RECLAIM YOUR BODY

THE ANTI-INFLAMMATORY DIET & LIFESTYLE PLAN FOR ENDOMETRIOSIS, PCOS, IBS, AND CHRONIC PAIN

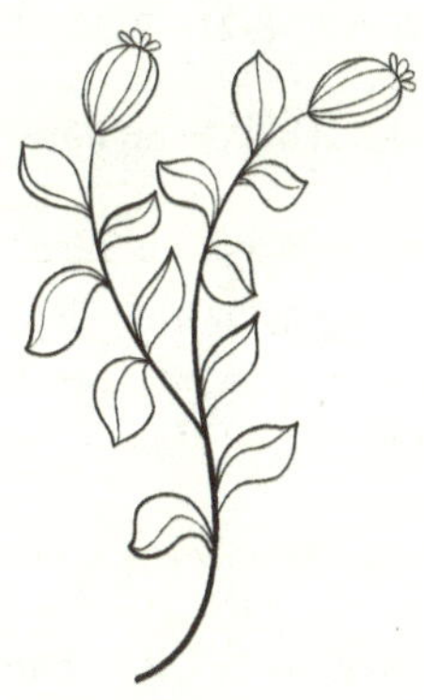

JOANNA BOROV

ISBN: 979-8-218-92120-0

Published by Joanna Borov

Illustrations by Natalia Tutanova
Cover design by Onur Burc
Interior formatting by Dawn Black
Back cover photograph by Nishelle Marie (@nishellemariephoto)

Printed in the United States of America.

WHAT EXPERTS ARE SAYING

"This book captures so much of what women with endometriosis and chronic illness suffer with, but struggle to define. It offers clear, actionable and compassionate advice that allows a reader to reapproach the relationship with their body and their environment - a valuable adjunct to holistic endometriosis care."

Amanda Chu, MD, FACOG
Minimally Invasive Gynecologic Surgeon and Endometriosis Specialist

"Women with chronic inflammatory conditions need validation first and foremost. Being heard and understood is often the first step toward healing. This book does exactly that — it validates women's experiences while empowering them with knowledge and tools to take control of their health."

— Marjorie Maye Mamsaang, DO
Doctor of Osteopathic Medicine; Board Certified in Physical Medicine and Rehabilitation; Board Certified in Physical Medicine & Rehabilitation and Sports Medicine,
Expert in Women's Sexual Health and Pelvic Pain

"Reclaim Your Body" is a valuable complement to medical care, offering women emotional support and motivation to take a conscious and proactive approach to their health. The author authentically and thoughtfully describes the experience of living with chronic illness, while maintaining a clear distinction between personal experience and medical treatment.

— Dariusz Zaryjewski, MD
Gynecologist & Endometriosis Specialist

"Reclaim Your Body speaks to women who have been dismissed, overwhelmed, or made to feel responsible for their pain. As both an endometriosis patient and a licensed acupuncturist, I deeply appreciate Joanna's compassionate, evidence-informed approach —one that supports the nervous system, reduces inflammation, and restores trust in the body without fear or false promises."

— Winnie Chan, L.Ac., MPA
Licensed Acupuncturist & Endometriosis Acupuncture Specialist

"Too many women live for years with symptoms that are minimized, misunderstood, or fragmented across the healthcare system. *Reclaim Your Body* offers an accessible guide to understanding inflammation, hormones, and the everyday practices that can help women feel more connected to and supported by their bodies."

— Shannon Cohn
Award-winning filmmaker, director and producer of the documentaries *Endo What?* and *Below the Belt,* and advocate for endometriosis awareness

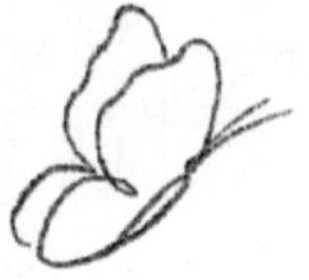

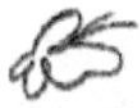

To Sarah Austin —

your bravery in honoring Trinity's pain has lit a path for millions of women.
When I reached out to thank you, I found a friend — someone who fights so others don't suffer alone.

This book is dedicated to you, and to every girl and woman who deserves to live without pain.

With all my love,
Joanna

*"We delight in the beauty of the butterfly,
but rarely admit the changes it has gone through
to achieve that beauty."*

TABLE OF CONTENTS

YOU DON'T HAVE TO GO THROUGH THIS ALONE

Living with chronic inflammation or conditions such as endometriosis can often feel isolating.

Many women spend years searching for answers, navigating conflicting advice, medical uncertainty, and the emotional weight of persistent symptoms.

Before we go any further, it is important to say something clearly: no illness is simply the result of not listening to your body or managing stress well enough. Chronic conditions are complex and influenced by many factors, including genetics, immune function, environmental exposures, and access to medical care. Emotional wellbeing and lifestyle habits can influence health, but they are only part of a much larger picture.

For this reason, healing is rarely a journey that should be taken alone.

Many women benefit from a team-based approach, where different professionals contribute their expertise. Depending on individual needs, this support network may include:

- physicians or endometriosis specialists
- registered dietitians or nutritionists
- pelvic floor physical therapists
- psychologists or therapists
- integrative practitioners such as acupuncturists

Support from community and other women living with similar conditions can also be incredibly valuable.

At the same time, living with a chronic condition can sometimes reveal that support does not always come from the places we initially expected. Friends, family members, or even healthcare providers may not always fully understand the experience of chronic illness. Yet many women also discover support in unexpected places — new communities, compassionate professionals, or people who simply choose to listen and stand beside them.

The lifestyle practices discussed in this book—such as nutrition, stress regulation, sleep, and nervous system support—can be valuable tools that support overall wellbeing. However, they are not a replacement for medical care, and they work best when integrated with guidance from qualified healthcare professionals.

Most importantly, remember that you deserve support, compassion, and partnership in your health journey. No one should have to navigate chronic illness alone.

PART I

UNDERSTANDING YOUR BODY

CHAPTER 1

LIVING WITH CHRONIC ILLNESS

Chronic illness reveals one undeniable truth: health is everything. When it's compromised, even ordinary tasks feel heavy, achievements lose impact, and joy becomes difficult to access. Physical symptoms don't stay in the body — they change how we think, feel, and relate to ourselves. Pain can be loud, but fatigue, anxiety, and hormonal instability are quiet weights that shape daily life and slowly erode confidence.

When I was first diagnosed with endometriosis, I didn't even know what it was. I felt embarrassed — how could a condition so severe be completely unfamiliar to me? I expected answers to bring relief, and at first they did. Finally, I wasn't imagining my pain. It wasn't "normal," or "just part of being a woman." But then I learned there was no cure, and the relief turned into dread. It felt like a lifetime sentence my body wouldn't allow me to escape.

For a year, I followed what I was told was the solution: hormonal medication. It didn't help. I chose surgery next, convinced that this was the real fix. I believed that once it was over, I would just feel better — that my body would reward me for enduring the procedure. The surgery lasted over six hours, yet I expected to bounce back in days. I wanted immediate results, the quick path to wellness. But chronic illness doesn't respond to impatience. It requires slow adaptation, not force.

Medication and surgery can be essential, but they don't create lasting healing on their own. I learned this the hard way. I had worked as a fashion model for years and assumed I was healthy because I was thin and active. I exercised constantly — not realizing that pushing the body into exhaustion isn't the same as caring for it. I ate what I believed was a "clean diet," but not one designed to support hormones, gut health, or inflammation. I was doing a lot for my health — but not what my body truly needed.

The shift began with mindset. How we think about our symptoms influences how we heal from them. The story we tell ourselves — whether we see our body as weak, unreliable, or burdensome — affects both our biology and our behavior. When I stopped demanding perfection and started listening without judgment, everything changed. Healing became a partnership, not a battle.

An anti-inflammatory lifestyle isn't restrictive — it's freeing. At first, it does require letting go of comfort foods, habits, or conveniences that inflame the body. It requires nuance in social settings, reading menus differently, explaining choices to others. But over time, these choices become empowering. What looks like sacrifice becomes self-respect. The joy of waking up without pain is greater than the pleasure of any processed snack or glass of wine. The reward is not perfection — it's relief.

People have told me, "Your life must be so miserable — you can't eat anything fun." But the truth is the opposite. I've discovered the joy of living without bloating, without monthly agony, without emotional chaos driven by inflammation. If I didn't have endometriosis, I would still choose this lifestyle — to protect my health, to age slower, to think more clearly, and to feel more like myself.

Do I still get symptoms? Yes — but they no longer control my life. That is healing.

Wellness is not simply eating less sugar or swapping pasta for broccoli. It's finding balance between protein, fiber, fats, micronutrients, and the needs of your microbiome. It's learning that gut health influences mood, hormones, immunity, and energy — that digestion is the physical foundation of mental clarity.

More than two-thirds of Americans experience frequent gastrointestinal symptoms (AbbVie Global Gastrointestinal Health Survey, 2022). Globally, over 40% live with chronic digestive conditions such as IBS or constipation (Sperber et al., 2021). Digestive disorders are no longer rare — they are the norm. But "common" doesn't mean "normal."

Healing requires supporting the gut, calming inflammation, and reconnecting with the body. And that is why I created **The 30-Day Healing Reset** — a practical, flexible plan designed to reduce inflammation, nourish digestive health, balance hormones, and support emotional well-being. It is not a diet. It is not a challenge. It is a reset — a return to what the body needs to thrive.

This Reset is about shifting identity: from pushing through symptoms to caring for yourself with awareness. From depending on quick fixes to building habits that feel sustainable. From fighting the body to working with it.

When we choose nourishment over restriction, patience over pressure, and awareness over frustration, we begin a lifelong relationship with our body — one rooted in trust.

Every choice you make for your health is an act of love toward yourself.

THE INVISIBLE WEIGHT

Chronic illness doesn't always begin with pain. Sometimes it starts as uncertainty — a whisper that something isn't right, even when test results say everything is "normal." Many women are conditioned to believe that fatigue, cramps, bloating, mood swings, and digestive discomfort are simply part of being female. We're taught to endure discomfort rather than question it.

My symptoms began quietly. During my cycle, I would feel a heavy fatigue that didn't match my lifestyle. I could somehow tolerate pain, but exhaustion was debilitating. Some days, I couldn't get out of bed without feeling like my body was made of concrete. This wasn't laziness, and it wasn't weakness. But at the time, I didn't understand that. I told myself to push harder, to ignore the whispers.

Chronic illness is often invisible. Symptoms overlap across systems: skin reactions, digestive distress, hormonal chaos, headaches, joint pain, anxiety, insomnia. They're treated separately in medical settings, even though they are deeply connected inside the body. When nothing shows up on scans or lab results, we begin to question ourselves. Self-doubt becomes the first wound.

Women carry this burden disproportionately. Almost 80% of autoimmune conditions occur in women. Writer and physician Dr. Gabor Maté explores how chronic illness often develops in people who silence their needs, suppress emotions, or prioritize others over themselves (Maté, 2003; 2022). Illness becomes a language — the body's final attempt to be heard.

Chronic conditions often do not travel alone. Endometriosis, IBS, migraines, thyroid disorders, fibromyalgia, histamine issues — they cluster not because the body is broken, but because it is overwhelmed. Chronic illness doesn't arrive suddenly. It is the buildup of years of unmet needs.

For a long time, I resented my body. I viewed it as unpredictable and fragile. I tried to control it with stricter routines, harsher diets, more force. But healing didn't begin until I stopped fighting and started listening. When I treated my body as an ally rather than a problem to fix, I gained insight. I could finally see what worsened symptoms and what soothed them.

Some days, healing means movement. Other days, rest is the most therapeutic choice you can make. True recovery requires flexibility, not discipline. It requires knowing when to act and when to allow. The goal is not to do more — it's to respond wisely.

Chronic illness teaches a new definition of productivity. A meaningful day may involve fewer tasks but more honesty with yourself. Healing isn't linear. There will be flares, pauses, progress, grief, clarity. This is not failure — it's rhythm.

Your body is not against you. It has been protecting you in the only way it knows how.

THE SPOON THEORY – UNDERSTANDING ENERGY AS A LIMITED RESOURCE

If you live with chronic illness, you may already know The Spoon Theory — a metaphor created by writer Christine Miserandino to describe what it feels like to move through the world with limited energy. In her story, she explains that each day begins with a certain number of "spoons." Each spoon represents a unit of energy.

Healthy people often have enough spoons to spend freely, without planning. But for those living with chronic illness or inflammation, energy is finite. Every activity — getting up, working, cooking, socializing, even answering a message — costs a spoon. When spoons run out, the body doesn't just feel tired; it enters a state of depletion that can trigger pain, fatigue, or inflammatory flares.

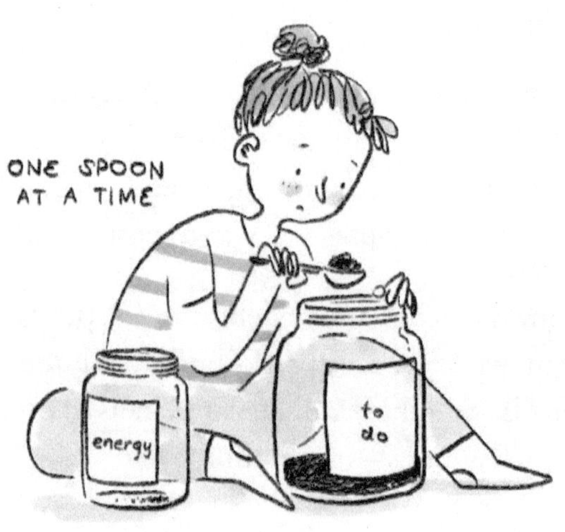

The Spoon Theory teaches something often overlooked: managing energy is a form of self-respect. Some days, you may start with ten spoons. Other days, you may wake up with only three. The goal isn't to push through, but to recognize capacity and honor it. This isn't weakness — it's wisdom.

This awareness naturally changes how you live. You begin to choose what matters, instead of doing what is expected. You start valuing rest as much as productivity. You begin letting go of people or commitments that drain you more than they nourish you. Protecting your energy becomes an act of healing.

Instead of trying to live like someone with unlimited spoons, you build a life that works with your capacity, not against it. That is healing in its most practical form.

WHY THIS BOOK?

This book was created through both research and lived experience — through years of experimenting, learning, and gradually discovering what actually supports healing. For a long time, I believed that "taking medication and eating healthy" were enough. Eventually I learned that they addressed only part of my reality. Healing wasn't just about what I consumed, but also about what I encountered daily: stress hormones still active in my nervous system, inflammatory ingredients hidden in common foods, poor sleep habits, environmental toxins, and emotional tension stored in my body.

I needed a complete approach, not fragmented advice. I needed to understand how the gut affects hormones, how stress fuels inflammation, how sleep impacts immunity, how movement can either heal or deplete, and how mindset influences every part of the healing process. Only when I saw the full picture did change become lasting.

If you're reading this, you may be on a similar path. Perhaps you've experienced chronic fatigue, bloating, pain, breakouts, or mood changes that don't make sense. Maybe you've been told your symptoms are "normal," or that you simply need to manage them. Or maybe you're simply ready to feel clearer, lighter, and more connected to your body — without obsessing, restricting, or guessing.

This book is for you if:

- You live with a chronic condition such as endometriosis, PCOS, IBS, Crohn's disease, or autoimmune symptoms.
- You've tried medications, diets, or supplements without lasting relief.
- You are tired of short-term fixes and want sustainable change.
- You believe (or are open to believing) that emotional and mental well-being affect physical health.
- You want practical guidance — not vague theories — to support your daily life.
- You want a lifestyle that feels nourishing rather than restrictive.

This is not a weight-loss book. Many people with chronic illness struggle to lose weight because inflammation disrupts hormones, gut balance, metabolism, and energy. If weight changes happen here, they happen because the body finds balance. Sustainable weight loss still requires a calorie deficit, but it becomes easier when inflammation is reduced and the body is supported instead of stressed.

Healing is the priority. When inflammation calms, digestion improves, and hormones stabilize, the body often lets go of what it no longer needs. This may include excess weight, but it may also include fatigue, joint pain, brain fog, or emotional heaviness. The most meaningful transformation isn't external. It's the return of clarity, energy, and trust.

As your gut heals and blood sugar stabilizes, something else shifts: your relationship with yourself. A calm nervous system and balanced digestion often bring emotional stability and sharper intuition. When the body isn't in defense mode, you can hear yourself clearly. You start choosing foods because they feel right, not because a rule tells you to. You move from control to awareness, from discipline to embodiment.

By the end of this book, you will understand:

- how inflammation develops and affects the body,
- how food, stress, and lifestyle contribute to symptoms,
- how to reduce inflammation through nutrition and mindset,
- how to nourish gut health and hormonal balance,
- how to build routines that support long-term healing.

Most importantly, you'll rebuild trust with your body — the foundation of sustainable wellness.

A note on medical care:

This book is intended for educational and informational purposes only. It is not a substitute for medical advice, diagnosis, or treatment. Every body is different, and healing is not one-size-fits-all. Always consult with a qualified healthcare professional before making changes to medications, supplements, or treatment plans — especially if you are managing a chronic condition. This book is meant to support your healing journey, not replace personalized medical care.

CHAPTER 2

WHAT IS INFLAMMATION

Inflammation is the body's defense mechanism — an intelligent, protective response designed to help us heal. When you get a cut, catch a virus, or experience injury, the immune system sends inflammatory cells to repair damage and fight invaders. This short-term (acute) inflammation is essential. The redness or swelling after an injury is your immune system actively protecting you (Medzhitov, 2008).

The problem arises when inflammation doesn't resolve. **Chronic inflammation** occurs when the immune system stays activated long after the original trigger has passed. Instead of repairing the body, it begins damaging healthy tissue. This low-grade, ongoing inflammation fuels pain, fatigue, digestive issues, and a wide range of diseases (Furman et al., 2019).

Chronic inflammation has been linked to:

- heart disease,
- diabetes,
- autoimmune conditions,
- arthritis,

- chronic digestive problems,
- hormonal imbalances,
- metabolic disorders,
- and even certain cancers (Furman et al., 2019).

It doesn't always show up as dramatic illness. Often it appears as everyday symptoms: bloating, brain fog, stubborn weight shifts, irritability, fatigue, skin flare-ups, or sleep disruption. Many people learn to tolerate these symptoms, not realizing they are early messages from the immune system.

Modern living fuels inflammation. The immune system becomes activated not only by infection or injury, but also by:

- processed foods and inflammatory oils,
- refined sugars and artificial additives,
- chronic stress and emotional suppression,
- sedentary habits or extreme exercise,
- poor sleep,
- environmental pollutants,
- and microbiome imbalance.

The mind and body are inseparable — emotional stress activates the same pathways as physical stress. The immune system listens to both (Rea et al., 2021).

The good news is this: inflammation is not an enemy to defeat — it's a signal to interpret. When we identify what the body is responding to, and support it through food, lifestyle, and emotional care, inflammation begins to quiet. Healing doesn't require fighting. It requires understanding.

CHAPTER 3

HOW CHRONIC INFLAMMATION SHOWS UP

Unlike a swollen injury or a fever, chronic inflammation doesn't always reveal itself through obvious signs. It can hide beneath subtle, persistent discomfort that we often dismiss as everyday stress, aging, or "just being a woman."

One of the most common — and overlooked — signs is persistent fatigue. When the immune system is continuously active, it consumes energy that should be available for living, thinking, and creating. What feels like unexplained tiredness or brain fog may be the body struggling to manage inflammation (Furman et al., 2019). Most people feel afternoon fatigue. I felt a shutdown. Around 3 PM my body would suddenly become dense and unresponsive, as if someone had turned down the dial on my energy. I'd lie on the sofa, whispering "two minutes," hoping the heaviness would pass. But two minutes often slipped into an hour. And on too many days, I'd cancel plans I was actually excited about — not because I changed my mind, but because my body simply quit on me. I eventually shifted my whole life around that collapse. I started waking up extremely early, trying to squeeze productivity into the morning hours, just in case the afternoon disappeared again.

Digestive issues are another major clue. Bloating, cramping, constipation, diarrhea, food sensitivities, or heaviness after meals signal a stressed gut. Because much of the immune system resides in the intestines, inflammation in the gut can affect hormones, mood, skin, metabolism, and immunity (Rea et al., 2021).

For many women, these symptoms quietly shape their entire day. A friend once told me she could describe every public bathroom near her office building because her IBS forced her to plan her schedule around proximity to a toilet. She never ate breakfast before meetings. She always chose an aisle seat "just in case." From the outside, she looked like the organized, high-performing woman who "has it all together." Inside, her gut dictated every decision.

If you find yourself planning your life around bathrooms, stretchy waistbands, avoiding certain restaurants, or calculating how far you'll be from home, that isn't you being dramatic. It's your body asking for attention — and it deserves to be heard.

Skin changes often reflect internal inflammation. Acne, rashes, hives, puffiness, or eczema can be linked to deeper immune responses. Joint pain, muscle aches, and headaches may also stem from inflammatory pathways rather than injury. I remember a period when I was under intense stress and tension, and suddenly I developed severe eczema on my eyelids. My skin was red, irritated, and painfully dry — and I couldn't figure out why. I spent hours researching creams, allergies, detergents, makeup ingredients, anything that could be causing it. Nothing made sense. Only later did I realize it wasn't a surface issue at all. It was my endometriosis and overall inflammation expressing themselves through my skin, amplified by stress and hormonal imbalance.

Skin doesn't flare "for no reason." It reacts to internal chaos long before we understand the message.

Inflammation influences emotional patterns as well. Anxiety, irritability, low mood, and difficulty concentrating have been associated with inflammatory markers, especially when the gut–brain axis is disrupted (Rea et al., 2021). Even weight changes — whether stubborn gain or sudden loss — can signal inflammatory and metabolic imbalance (Furman et al., 2019).

These symptoms are often treated individually, yet they share a common source. This is why chronic illness can feel sudden. Disease rarely appears "out of nowhere." The body often communicates through whispers long before it reaches a breaking point. Chronic inflammation is the quiet spark beneath many conditions we address only once they become fire.

Long before modern medicine, Hippocrates taught that the body, mind, emotions, and environment are inseparable — that imbalance in one area inevitably affects the whole person. For centuries, healing was viewed as a unified process.

That changed in the 17th century, when philosopher René Descartes introduced the concept of mind–body dualism, separating thought from physiology. This idea shaped Western medicine for centuries, leading practitioners to treat symptoms in isolation rather than as part of a connected system.

Today, modern science brings us full circle. Psychoneuroimmunology, the gut–brain axis, and inflammation research all confirm what ancient medicine already understood: the mind and body are inseparable. Stress, immunity, digestion, hormones, and emotion constantly influence one another. The body has never been divided — it speaks as an interconnected whole.

CHAPTER 4

THE HIDDEN ROOTS OF INFLAMMATION

Modern illness rarely begins with dramatic symptoms. It builds quietly, accumulating through lifestyle habits, environmental exposure, and unresolved stress. Chronic inflammation often starts long before any diagnosis — in the daily routines we overlook, the foods we normalize, the rest we skip, and the emotions we suppress.

It begins subtly. Days fueled by processed convenience foods, mornings rushed without nourishment, evenings spent overstimulated but exhausted. Sleep that never quite repairs us. Stress that lingers in muscles we never fully relax. The body adapts to these patterns, but adaptation is not the same as thriving.

Inflammation is not only a biological response — it is the body's reaction to imbalance. When we consistently eat foods the body doesn't recognize, ignore emotional stress, suppress symptoms, or deprive ourselves of rest, the immune system becomes overactive. It stops responding only to infection or injury and begins reacting to everyday life.

Stress plays a significant role. Stress itself is not harmful; it is part of being alive. What damages the body is **chronic stress without recovery** — the unexhaled breath, the lack of reset after daily tension. When stress hormones stay elevated, the immune system remains on alert, and inflammation becomes ongoing rather than adaptive.

Not all inflammatory triggers are obvious. Some are universal — chronic stress, poor sleep, nutrient deficiencies. Others accumulate slowly: environmental toxins, endocrine disruptors, hormonal imbalance, overuse of NSAIDs or antibiotics, or years of eating inflammatory foods. Healing must therefore begin with what we encounter most consistently: nourishment, rest, movement, and emotional regulation.

Inflammation is not sudden. It is a gradual echo of imbalance. It is the body's final attempt to communicate after whispers have gone unheard. When we respond with care instead of control, the body no longer has to shout through pain. It softens — and healing becomes possible.

HORMONAL IMBALANCE – WHEN THE BODY'S MESSENGERS LOSE THEIR RHYTHM

Hormones are chemical messengers that direct nearly every system in the body. They influence metabolism, mood, pain perception, gut motility, inflammation, sleep, and immune communication. When these messengers drift out of balance, the entire internal ecosystem becomes reactive.

For women with endometriosis, PCOS, IBS, thyroid disorders, or chronic inflammation, hormonal imbalance is not a surface issue — it is a core driver of symptoms.

Hormones and inflammation form a loop:
when hormones destabilize, inflammation rises — and when inflammation rises, hormones destabilize further.
Breaking this loop is essential for healing.

ESTROGEN DOMINANCE (ABSOLUTE OR RELATIVE)

Estrogen becomes dominant when the body has too much estrogen, too little progesterone, or difficulty clearing estrogen through the liver and bowels.
This imbalance can amplify:

- pelvic and menstrual pain
- breast tenderness
- migraines
- fluid retention and bloating
- mood swings
- histamine sensitivity

Estrogen activates mast cells and prostaglandins, both involved in the inflammatory cascade of endometriosis and PMS. When estrogen is not efficiently metabolized, symptoms intensify.

INSULIN RESISTANCE

Frequent glucose spikes keep insulin elevated, which increases systemic inflammation and disrupts ovarian and adrenal hormones. Early signs often include:

- energy crashes
- cravings (especially for sugar or carbs)
- irritability
- stubborn weight around the waist
- brain fog

Stabilizing blood sugar is one of the most effective ways to reduce inflammation and hormonal chaos.

THYROID DYSREGULATION

Thyroid hormones regulate metabolic rate, temperature, gut motility, and energy production.
When the thyroid slows, women often experience:

- constipation
- cold hands and feet
- fatigue and brain fog
- hair shedding
- low mood

Because autoimmune thyroid disorders like Hashimoto's are common in women with chronic inflammation, supporting the immune system and reducing inflammatory load naturally improves thyroid resilience.

CORTISOL MISMATCH (STRESS AXIS DYSREGULATION)

Cortisol follows a daily rhythm — high in the morning, lower at night.
When this rhythm becomes distorted by chronic stress, symptoms shift depending on the pattern:

High cortisol:

- anxiety
- insomnia
- digestive shutdown
- wired–tired exhaustion

Low cortisol:

- morning heaviness
- apathy
- low stress tolerance
- afternoon crashes

Both patterns disrupt blood sugar, sex hormones, thyroid function, and immune balance.

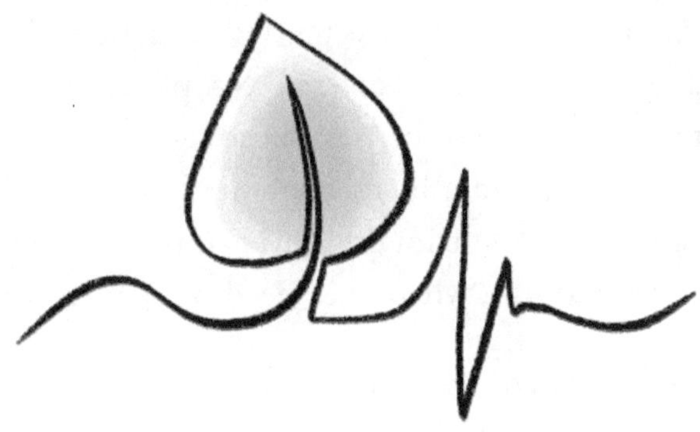

HOW TO BEGIN RESTORING HORMONAL BALANCE

These changes create a foundation for hormonal regulation:

1. Stabilize insulin with balanced meals:

Always include **protein + fiber + healthy fats** to prevent glucose spikes and crashes.

2. Support estrogen metabolism:

- cruciferous vegetables (broccoli, cauliflower, arugula, cabbage)
- bitter foods (dandelion, radicchio, lemon water)
- hydration
- daily bowel movements
  These help the liver and gut clear estrogen efficiently.

Hydration plays an important role in hormone balance, digestion, and the body's ability to eliminate excess estrogen efficiently. Adequate fluid intake supports the liver, digestive tract, and lymphatic system, all of which help reduce inflammatory burden. A simple approach is to drink water consistently throughout the day rather than waiting until you feel depleted. Simple additions such as a pinch of mineral salt, fresh berries, sliced lemon, or cucumber can enhance both flavor and mineral content, making hydration more enjoyable and easier to maintain. This can be especially refreshing during warmer months, when fluid needs may increase.

While whole fruits are encouraged, fruit juices are more concentrated in natural sugars and may not be ideal for daily consumption for some individuals. Enjoying juices occasionally—such as green juice or pomegranate juice once or twice per week—can be a balanced approach. Another option is to dilute juices, such as cranberry juice, with water to reduce sugar concentration while still enjoying their flavor.

3. Restore circadian rhythm:

- morning light exposure
- dim evenings
- consistent sleep

This regulates cortisol, thyroid function, and reproductive hormones.

4. Choose movement that builds, not drains:

Gentle strength training + daily walking improves insulin sensitivity and lowers inflammation without overstimulating the nervous system.

GUT IMBALANCE – LEAKY GUT, DYSBIOSIS, AND CANDIDA

Gut imbalance begins when there is a disruption in the microbiome — the ecosystem of bacteria, yeast, and microorganisms living in the intestines. In a healthy gut, beneficial bacteria help digest food, produce vitamins, regulate hormones, and maintain a protective gut lining. But when harmful bacteria or yeast begin to dominate, this balance is lost, leading to inflammation and systemic symptoms (Belkaid & Hand, 2014).

More than 70% of the immune system resides in the gut, which means that microbiome imbalance has direct effects on immune function, hormonal balance, and inflammatory pathways (Round & Mazmanian, 2009). Antibiotics, alcohol, chronic stress, low-fiber diets, high-sugar intake, environmental toxins, and certain medications weaken the gut barrier and reduce beneficial bacteria. As the intestinal lining becomes more permeable, undigested particles and bacterial toxins can enter the bloodstream — a condition commonly known as **leaky gut**. The immune system perceives these particles as threats, triggering chronic inflammation.

Gut imbalance doesn't always show up as digestive symptoms. While bloating, gas, cramping, or constipation are common, others experience:

- fatigue,
- brain fog,
- joint pain,

- stubborn weight changes,
- skin rashes or acne,
- recurrent infections,
- mood instability or anxiety.

The gut communicates continuously with the brain through the **gut–brain axis**, which means dysbiosis can influence emotional state, stress response, and cognitive function (Carabotti et al., 2015). A balanced microbiome supports a calm mood and clear thinking, while imbalance fuels inflammation, hormonal disruption, and emotional distress.

CANDIDA OVERGROWTH – WHEN YEAST TAKES OVER

One of the most frequent causes of dysbiosis is **Candida overgrowth** — an excessive growth of a yeast that naturally lives in the gut, mouth, and vaginal area. Normally, beneficial bacteria keep Candida in check. But when the microbiome is disrupted — through antibiotic use, high sugar intake, hormonal changes, stress, or nutrient deficiencies — Candida can multiply and penetrate the gut lining. This contributes to systemic inflammation and immune activation (Iliev & Leonardi, 2017).

Candida overgrowth may cause symptoms such as:

- bloating after meals,
- sugar cravings,
- fatigue,
- brain fog,
- recurrent yeast infections,
- sinus congestion,
- skin issues,
- oral thrush.

Because Candida produces toxins that irritate the gut lining, it can worsen leaky gut and intensify inflammatory responses. The goal of healing is not to eliminate yeast entirely — it is a natural part of the microbiome — but to **restore balance** so it does not dominate.

RESTORING GUT BALANCE – FOUNDATIONS OF HEALING

Healing the gut is not about strict dieting or extreme elimination. It is a process of nourishment and consistency. A healthy gut requires three key steps:

1. Feed beneficial bacteria

Choose whole, fiber-rich, plant foods that support microbiome diversity: vegetables, leafy greens, seeds, legumes, and moderate fruit. Reduce refined sugar, alcohol, and processed foods that feed harmful microbes.

2. Support Microbial Diversity

A healthy gut is like a balanced garden:
it needs **good bacteria (probiotics)** *and* the **food that helps them grow (prebiotics).**

Prebiotics
These are types of fiber that **feed beneficial bacteria**, helping them grow stronger.
They are found in foods such as:

- garlic
- leeks
- asparagus
- oats
- flaxseed

Probiotics

These are **live beneficial bacteria** that help increase the number of healthy microbes in the gut.

They are found in fermented foods such as:

- sauerkraut
- kimchi
- miso
- coconut yogurt

Some individuals may also benefit from **targeted probiotic supplements**, especially after antibiotic use or chronic digestive problems (Hemarajata & Versalovic, 2013).

3. Protect and repair the gut lining

Nutrients such as zinc, glutamine, and omega-3 fatty acids aid tissue repair. Hydration, balanced meals, and mindful eating reduce digestive strain.

Additionally:

- Natural antifungals like oregano, caprylic acid, garlic, and pau d'arco may assist Candida balance — but should be used gradually to avoid strong "die-off" reactions.
- Stress management is essential. Chronic cortisol imbalance disrupts gut motility and microbiota (Carabotti et al., 2015). Practices such as diaphragmatic breathing, meditation, tapping, or gentle yoga can regulate the gut–brain axis.

A healthy gut is more than the absence of symptoms. It is a feeling of lightness, clarity, emotional steadiness, and reliable digestion. The microbiome influences how we think, feel, and heal. Supporting it is one of the most powerful steps toward reducing inflammation and restoring vitality.

MITOCHONDRIA – THE HIDDEN ENGINE OF ENERGY AND HEALING

There are days when exhaustion feels bone-deep — a heaviness no amount of sleep can relieve. Many people assume fatigue is caused by hormones, stress, or lack of sleep, and these do play a role. But beneath them lies a more fundamental factor: **the mitochondria** — the tiny organelles responsible for generating energy (ATP) in every cell.

When mitochondria function optimally, we experience mental clarity, stable mood, and physical energy. When they slow down, fatigue, brain fog, and weakness appear. For those with chronic inflammation or hormonal imbalance, mitochondrial dysfunction is a critical but often overlooked piece of the puzzle.

Inflammation changes the environment in which mitochondria operate. When the immune system is chronically activated, it releases free radicals and inflammatory cytokines that impair mitochondrial membranes. These free radicals deplete antioxidants quickly, creating **oxidative stress**, which damages the enzymes needed for ATP production.

As mitochondrial function declines, the body limits energy to conserve resources. Metabolism slows, muscles feel heavy, cognitive function becomes sluggish, and recovery after activity takes longer. Many people describe it as feeling "wired but tired" — anxious, overstimulated, yet unable to generate real energy. This is not a lack of motivation. It is cellular exhaustion.

Key contributors to mitochondrial dysfunction include:

- oxidative stress from chronic inflammation,
- nutrient depletion (loss of magnesium, B vitamins, iron, CoQ10),

- hormonal imbalance (especially thyroid and cortisol dysregulation),
- microbiome imbalance,
- chronic infection or immune activation.

Signs of mitochondrial depletion often include:

- fatigue not improved by sleep,
- brain fog or forgetfulness,
- muscle weakness after minimal exertion,
- anxiety with physical exhaustion,
- cold hands and feet,
- slow recovery after illness or exercise.

Restoring mitochondrial function requires creating conditions in which energy can be produced naturally. This includes:

- replenishing key nutrients such as CoQ10 (especially ubiquinol), magnesium, iron, and B vitamins;
- stabilizing blood sugar through balanced meals rich in whole foods;
- gentle movement that increases oxygen without overexertion;
- prioritizing sleep, particularly before midnight, when mitochondrial repair is most active;
- reducing inflammatory foods and environmental toxins.

As inflammation decreases, mitochondria return to balance, and energy begins to flow again — not as a forced effort, but as a natural expression of a supported body. Fatigue becomes less mysterious when we understand it at the cellular level. Healing begins not with caffeine or adrenaline, but with nourishment, oxygen, and cellular restoration.

THE LYMPHATIC SYSTEM – CLEARING THE PATH FOR RECOVERY

Most people focus on blood circulation, yet the lymphatic system is just as crucial — especially for those experiencing chronic inflammation. If the bloodstream delivers nutrients and oxygen, the lymphatic system is responsible for cleaning up what's left behind. It removes waste, inflammatory molecules, toxins, and cellular debris, helping the immune system function efficiently (Olszewski, 2003).

Unlike the circulatory system, the lymphatic system has **no pump**. It relies entirely on movement, breath, muscle contraction, and hydration to circulate. When lymph flow stagnates, waste remains in tissues longer than it should, creating an environment where inflammation accumulates. Symptoms of lymph stagnation often include:

- puffiness in the face or body,
- swollen fingers or ankles,
- bloating without weight gain,
- brain fog,
- heaviness in the body,
- tenderness near lymph nodes,
- chronic fatigue or recurring infections.

Chronic inflammation thickens lymph fluid and damages lymphatic vessel tone through inflammatory cytokines, further slowing circulation (Randolph et al., 2017). Sedentary behavior, dehydration, poor posture, and tight fascia also restrict lymph movement. Over time, this creates a cycle: inflammation slows lymph flow, and slow lymph flow perpetuates inflammation.

Supporting lymph health does not require extreme detoxes. It requires consistent habits that restore flow:

- daily movement such as walking, light stretching, yoga, or rebounding;
- deep diaphragmatic breathing, which acts as a natural lymph pump;
- mineral-rich hydration to prevent lymph fluid from thickening;
- gentle lymphatic massage or dry brushing;
- alternating warm and cool water in showers to stimulate vessels;
- loosening tight fascia through stretching or myofascial release.

In Eastern medicine, lymphatic stagnation is viewed as stagnation of energy — an emotional and physical blockage. Practices such as acupuncture, gua sha, cupping, and oil massage support fluid movement and energetic release (Lu et al., 2004; Sharma & Dash, 2017). When the body learns to release physical waste, it often releases emotional tension as well. Clarity follows flow.

Detailed instructions for dry brushing can be found in the appendix.

EASTERN MEDICINE, EMOTIONAL HEALTH, AND THE ENERGETIC BODY

Long before modern science could name hormones, neurotransmitters, or immune messengers, ancient systems of medicine recognized the connections between emotions, lifestyle, and physical health. While Western medicine traditionally separates body and mind, Eastern traditions such as Traditional Chinese Medicine (TCM) and Ayurveda view them as inseparable aspects of the same experience. Today, neuroscience and immunology increasingly support what these systems have taught for centuries.

Chronic stress does not only affect mood; it impacts digestion, immune function, pain perception, and hormonal regulation. The nervous system communicates directly with the immune system, meaning emotional suppression, unresolved conflict, or constant pressure can activate inflammatory pathways in the same way as injury or infection. This field of research, known as **psychoneuroimmunology**, demonstrates scientifically what holistic medicine has always understood: emotional health influences physical inflammation.

<u>Eastern medicine describes this concept through energy and flow.</u>

In **TCM**, illness is associated with stagnation — when Qi (vital energy) and bodily fluids stop moving freely. Stress, traumatic experiences, repressed emotions, and chronic fatigue are believed to obstruct flow, leading to pain, swelling, and imbalance. Techniques such as acupuncture, cupping, gua sha, and herbal therapy gently restore circulation, helping the body return to homeostasis. Modern research increasingly shows that these therapies influence inflammation, blood flow, and nervous system regulation.

In **Ayurveda**, the lymphatic system is called *rasa dhatu*, the first and most essential tissue of the body. It nourishes every other system, supports immunity, and is linked to emotional resilience. Ayurvedic practices such as **abhyanga** (warm oil massage), **garshana** (dry brushing), and herbal detoxification cleanse the lymph, calm the nervous system, and support inflammatory balance (Sharma & Dash, 2017). They are not extreme detoxes; they are nurturing, rhythmic forms of stimulation designed to reestablish flow.

While Eastern medicine uses metaphors of energy, Western science describes biochemical markers, neurotransmitters, cytokines, and hormones. Yet both are describing the same phenomenon from different perspectives. Emotional and physical inflammation coexist; neither is purely psychological nor purely biological. They are intertwined responses of a body trying to protect itself.

When we speak of "energy" in holistic healing, it can be understood biologically as:

- nervous system tone,
- mitochondrial output,
- blood circulation,
- lymph flow,
- hormone signaling,
- and microbiome communication.

These are the physical expressions of vitality. When they stagnate, we feel tired, heavy, anxious, or inflamed. When they move freely, we feel clear, calm, and energized.

Healing is not simply the removal of disease. It is the restoration of flow — biological, emotional, and energetic. Whether you call it **Qi, rasa (the nourishing fluid of the body), circulation, or nervous system regulation**, the principle is the same: health requires movement. Movement in the breath, the gut, the lymph, the mind, and in daily choices. Chronic illness is not only a disruption of cells, but a disruption of flow.

As inflammation quiets and flow returns, the body stops sounding alarms. It begins to trust you, and you begin to trust it. That is the foundation on which the Reset is built.

CHAPTER 5

THE 30-DAY HEALING RESET – A NEW FOUNDATION

Healing doesn't begin with strict rules, heavy discipline, or sudden change. It begins with understanding, and with a gentle shift in how you care for yourself. Many chronic conditions become overwhelming not because the body is weak, but because it has been fighting for too long without enough support. This Reset is not another diet or challenge. It is an invitation to create conditions in which your body can finally rest, repair, and rebuild.

The goal over the next 30 days is not perfection. It's consistency without pressure. You don't need to do everything at once, or feel motivated every day. You don't need flawless nutrition, strict routines, or high energy to participate. All you need is a willingness to treat your body like an ally — even if you don't fully trust it yet. Healing often begins before belief does.

This Reset is about nourishing your cells, calming inflammation, balancing the nervous system, supporting digestion, and gently shifting metabolism and hormones. The changes you make will be realistic, sustainable, and built to fit your life — not to control it. Small actions, repeated over time, change chemistry more effectively than intense efforts that you can't maintain.

The foundation of this Reset rests on four pillars:

- **Anti-inflammatory nutrition** that stabilizes blood sugar, supports the microbiome, and reduces immune activation.
- **Gentle daily movement** that stimulates circulation, oxygen flow, and lymphatic cleansing without exhausting the body.
- **Emotional and nervous system care**, because the body cannot repair when it feels unsafe.
- **Consistent sleep and circadian rhythms**, allowing real cellular repair to take place each night.

Instead of pushing your body to heal, you will give it permission to heal. Instead of forcing change, you will create the conditions for change to happen naturally. You aren't here to fight your symptoms. You're here to support the intelligence beneath them.

You don't have to be ready. You don't have to be sure. You simply have to begin.

Healing works best when each small step reinforces the next. The Reset is designed to build rhythm gently. You will eat in a way that reduces inflammation without feeling deprived, move in ways that support circulation without depletion, sleep in a way that rebuilds cellular energy, and create space for emotional release without force. These shifts may feel subtle at first, but subtle shifts create long-lasting change. They don't shock the body; they invite balance.

Throughout this Reset, you may notice moments of clarity, quieter symptoms, or a sense of steadiness returning. You may also experience fluctuations — occasional fatigue, digestive changes, or emotional sensitivity. These are not failures or setbacks. They are signs of the body reorganizing itself. Healing is not linear. It unfolds through adjustments, pauses, and gradual integration.

Think of this Reset not as "doing something to your body," but as **working with your body**. Instead of asking your body to perform, you will be asking it what it needs. What foods feel supportive? What pace feels sustainable? When does rest feel more productive than movement? When do you feel safe enough to let the nervous system settle? This kind of awareness makes healing more powerful than any supplement or diet alone.

You're not being asked to take control; you're being asked to create space for your body to use its intelligence. Every system — the gut, lymph, hormones, mitochondria, immune response — is already designed to heal. It simply needs the conditions to do so.

Over the next 30 days, you will gradually build a new foundation. You won't chase results. Instead, you'll learn how to support the body consistently so results arrive on their own timeline. You don't need to earn your way to health by effort or perfection. You already have everything required to heal; you are simply learning how to access it.

This Reset is the beginning of that relationship.

To begin the Reset, we start with the foundation that influences everything else: nourishment. Food is more than fuel; it shapes hormones, calms or aggravates inflammation, communicates with the immune system, and feeds the bacteria that support digestion and emotional balance. The goal of anti-inflammatory eating is not to remove joy from your plate. It is to choose foods that speak clearly to the body instead of confusing it with substances it doesn't recognize.

Instead of focusing on what you cannot eat, you will begin by giving your body what it has been missing. Many inflammatory foods only have such strong effects because the body is already depleted — of micronutrients, of fiber, of healthy fats, of amino acids, of antioxidants. When you restore nourishment, inflammation naturally loses its intensity. The body becomes less reactive. Digestion becomes less strained. Hormones become steadier. Sugar cravings quiet down not by force, but because your cells are finally receiving the building blocks they need.

Anti-inflammatory eating during this Reset emphasizes real food that comes without chemical manipulation. You will be choosing foods that stabilize blood sugar, support hormone detoxification, nourish your microbiome, and reduce oxidative stress. You're not controlling your body through food; you're communicating with it. You're offering nutrients that help it repair rather than merely survive.

You **can't lower inflammation while eating foods that trigger it**. That's why the first step of this Reset is **eliminating inflammatory and processed foods** and replacing them with options that support healing. This isn't about punishment or rigid dieting — it's about understanding that certain foods create stress in the body, and others calm it.

Once the inflammatory triggers are removed, we focus on nourishment. You learn what foods give you steady energy, what keeps digestion calm, and what helps your hormones stabilize. As the body begins to feel safe, inflammation drops, symptoms become more predictable, and cravings change naturally.

This Reset **is not temporary**. It teaches a way of eating you can maintain long term — not by perfection, but by choosing foods that support your gut, hormones, metabolism, and immune system. The more consistently you provide your body with the nutrients it needs, the easier it becomes to sustain results without restriction or obsessive rules.

You're not cutting foods to shrink yourself; you're clearing the noise so your body can function the way it's meant to.

Nutrition is only one pillar. Movement is another. Movement matters — but how you move matters even more. The goal is not to push through exhaustion or obsess over burning calories. With chronic inflammation, stress, and hormone imbalance, forcing the body to perform often backfires. Intense workouts on low energy days can elevate cortisol, worsen inflammation, and make symptoms more unpredictable. What supports healing is movement that builds strength, circulation, and resilience without overwhelming your system.

For women, especially those living with endometriosis, PCOS, IBS, or chronic pain, muscle strength is not optional — it's protective. Research shows that strength-training improves metabolic health, reduces inflammation, supports hormone balance, boosts insulin sensitivity, and helps maintain bone density over time. As Dr. Stacy Sims, one of the leading experts in female exercise physiology, explains, women who train for strength **and** power experience significantly better long-term health outcomes, particularly in metabolic and musculoskeletal function (Sims, *Train for Power, Not Just Strength*).

Strength-training a few times per week — using resistance bands, weights, or body-weight exercises — helps build muscle in a way that supports the nervous system instead of stressing it. On higher-energy days, you might choose more challenging workouts such as moderate weights, pilates, or interval training. On lower-energy days, the best choice may be a walk, gentle stretching, slow yoga, or simply letting your body rest without guilt.

Movement doesn't have to look like "exercise" to count. Daily life offers opportunities to support your body without stepping into a gym: taking the stairs instead of the elevator, walking instead of driving short distances, carrying groceries, standing while folding laundry, cleaning, dancing while cooking, or aiming for 20–30 minutes of walking spread throughout the day. These small, consistent choices improve circulation, lymphatic drainage, cellular energy, and mood — often more sustainably than intense workouts.

And on flare-up days, it is normal and healthy to do nothing. Pushing through severe pain, exhaustion, or inflammation can worsen symptoms and prolong recovery. Rest *is part of healing.* A supportive movement practice isn't defined by how hard you work, but by how well you listen. When movement is chosen with respect for your body's capacity, the body learns safety rather than survival — and safety is what allows inflammation to calm and healing to progress.

Rest is as important as nourishment and movement. The nervous system controls digestion, immune activity, hormone release, and inflammation. If the body believes it must stay alert, it cannot repair, even if you eat perfectly. Stress is not the enemy; the absence of recovery is. Creating small pockets of safety — through breath, boundaries, quiet, stillness, expression, or emotional honesty — is a form of medicine. When the nervous system softens, inflammation softens with it.

Finally, sleep becomes the part of your day where healing is most active. During deep sleep, mitochondria repair themselves, the brain detoxifies metabolic waste, hormones recalibrate, and tissues regenerate. You do not need perfect sleep to benefit. You only need to support your body's rhythms — dimming light in the evening, creating stillness before bed, honoring darkness at night, seeking sunlight in the morning. These small adjustments guide your body toward deeper sleep without forcing it.

Together, these four pillars — nourishment, movement, nervous system care, and sleep — create an environment in which inflammation begins to fade. Over the next 30 days, you will not focus on quick change. You will build a foundation that lasts far beyond this Reset. You are not trying to fix your body. You are learning how to support it so it can heal itself.

This book begins with understanding — because real change requires education first. If we want lasting healing, we need to know *why* things work, not just *what* to do. When we understand how inflammation develops, how hormones react to stress, and how food, sleep, movement, and the gut all influence each other, the choices we make become more intuitive. We no longer "force ourselves to follow a plan." We follow it because it finally makes sense.

Before we move into the Reset itself, the next chapters will give you the foundation: how inflammation affects chronic illness, how nutrition supports hormonal balance, why the gut matters, how stress impacts immunity, and why lifestyle habits create long-term change. Once these core pieces are clear, the Reset becomes not a restriction, but a logical progression — a way of eating and living that supports your body instead of fighting against it.

FROM INFLAMMATION TO BALANCE

Chronic illness often feels like a loss — loss of energy, loss of certainty, loss of who we used to be. But the truth beneath all symptoms is not loss. It is communication. Pain, fatigue, bloating, hormonal changes, brain fog — none of these are signs of a broken body. They are signals from a body asking for support.

Inflammation is not the enemy. It is the body's language when balance is missing. The immune system does not create symptoms to punish you; it creates them to protect you. It slows your energy when mitochondria are overwhelmed. It sends digestive distress when the gut lining is inflamed. It brings hormonal chaos when survival feels more urgent than reproduction. It asks you to pause, nourish, rebuild, and listen.

Health is not the absence of symptoms. It is the presence of connection. When we stop blaming our bodies and start understanding what they are asking for, healing becomes possible. Not because we force it, but because we stop resisting it.

Throughout this first part, you've learned that:

- inflammation is a physiological response, not a personal failure,
- the gut, lymphatic system, mitochondria, and nervous system all participate in healing,
- emotional and structural balance determine how the immune system behaves,
- the body is not unpredictable — it is deeply responsive to how you live, eat, move, and rest.

If illness can develop through small, repeated imbalances, then healing can develop through small, repeated acts of support. You do not need dramatic interventions to change your body. You only need consistency in giving it what it has been missing.

It took me a long time — years of trial and error — to understand what actually helped me and what triggered my flares. I had to learn how my body responded to stress, which foods and products to avoid, and which rituals became non-negotiable for my healing. Over time, something shifted. I became almost protective of my body instead of frustrated with it, and I grew passionate about sharing what I had learned so other women wouldn't have to suffer in silence. **And yes — I still have my off-routine days. Healing didn't make me perfect; it made me resilient.**

The next part of this book is where healing becomes practical. You will not fight your symptoms. You will not try to control your body. Instead, you will build the conditions for restoration — slowly, steadily, and without pressure. You will begin to eat, move, sleep, and live in ways that remind your body it is safe enough to heal.

Part II is not about striving for health. It is about returning to a relationship with your body that honors how hard it has been trying to protect you.

Healing begins not when we demand change, but when we finally listen.,

PART II

ELIMINATING THE TRIGGERS THAT INFLAME YOUR BODY

CHAPTER 6

THE TOXIC BURDEN: CHEMICALS THAT DISRUPT YOUR HORMONES

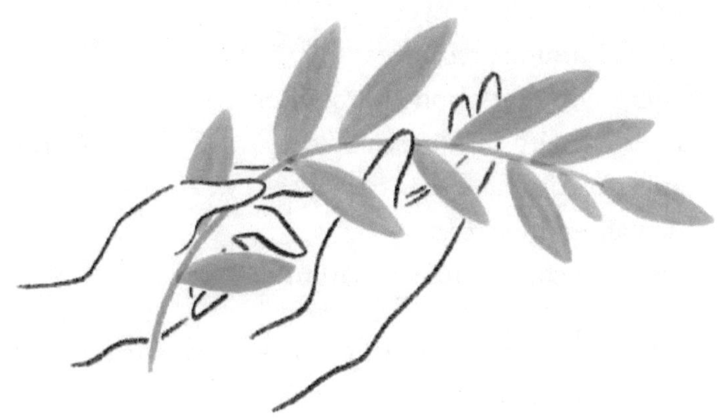

Chronic inflammation is not driven by food and stress alone. One of the most overlooked — yet powerful — contributors is daily exposure to endocrine-disrupting chemicals (EDCs). These compounds interfere with estrogen, progesterone, thyroid hormones, cortisol, insulin, and immune function. They accumulate quietly, often years before symptoms become visible, and they directly worsen conditions such as endometriosis, PCOS, IBS, hypothyroidism, and chronic fatigue.

The Endocrine Society, the World Health Organization, and leading research institutions classify EDCs as major contributors to hormone-related disorders, infertility, and chronic inflammatory diseases. These exposures often go unnoticed, but their effects do not. Reducing them significantly lowers your inflammatory load and gives your body more room to heal.

How Chemical Exposure Disrupts Hormones and Inflammation

Endocrine disruptors can:

- mimic natural estrogen
- block hormone receptors
- alter thyroid hormone production
- interfere with insulin sensitivity
- affect cortisol and the stress response
- damage gut bacteria
- promote chronic inflammation

Over time, this creates hormonal chaos — even when your bloodwork appears "normal." Many women discover that symptoms they blamed on stress, diet, or bad luck were actually fueled by daily chemical exposures hidden in products they use every day.

MAJOR ENDOCRINE DISRUPTORS AND WHAT RESEARCH SHOWS

Phthalates

Common in plastics, artificial fragrances, shampoos, lotions, nail polish, and household cleaning products. They can enter the body

through skin absorption, inhalation, and food stored in plastic. Once inside, they interfere with hormone receptors and alter estrogen and androgen balance.
Research: Phthalates worsen estrogen-driven inflammation and are associated with more severe cases of endometriosis and impaired fertility. *(Meeker et al., Human Reproduction Update, 2009)*

Bisphenol A (BPA)
Present in plastic bottles, food can linings, thermal receipts, and many plastic food containers. BPA leaches into food and beverages and remains biologically active once absorbed.
Research: BPA mimics estrogen, disrupts gut microbiome balance, and increases inflammatory responses linked to endometriosis and PCOS. *(Peretz et al., Reproductive Toxicology, 2014)*

PFAS ("Forever Chemicals")
Used in waterproof clothing, stain-resistant fabrics, take-out packaging, nonstick cookware, and fast-food wrappers. These compounds persist in the environment and accumulate in human tissues over time.
Research: PFAS exposure has been linked to thyroid dysfunction, fertility challenges, immune disruption, and inflammatory disorders. *(Sunderland et al., Environmental Science & Technology, 2019)*

Parabens
Found in cosmetics, lotions, shampoos, deodorants, and many "moisturizing" products. They readily penetrate the skin and are detectable in blood, urine, and reproductive tissue.
Research: Parabens act as weak estrogens and contribute to hormonal imbalance in estrogen-sensitive conditions. *(Boberg et al., Critical Reviews in Toxicology, 2010)*

Pesticides (e.g., Atrazine)
Present on conventionally farmed produce, grains, and contaminated water. These chemicals accumulate in soil and can persist on foods even after washing.
Research: Atrazine disrupts ovulation, alters estrogen activity, and interferes with reproductive hormone signaling. *(Hayes et al., Journal of Steroid Biochemistry, 2011)*

Dioxins & PCBs
Persistent industrial pollutants found in meat, dairy, and certain fish due to environmental accumulation. These compounds store in animal fat and then accumulate in human tissues through consumption.

Some research has linked persistent environmental pollutants such as dioxins and PCBs to inflammatory pathways involved in endometriosis and immune activation. (Rier et al., Toxicological Sciences, 2001)

Laboratory and animal studies suggest that certain environmental pollutants, including dioxins, may influence immune signaling and the development of endometriosis-like lesions. Some observational studies in humans have also reported higher levels of these compounds in individuals with endometriosis compared with control groups.

However, it is important to recognize that much of this research shows correlation rather than definitive causation. Large randomized controlled trials demonstrating that environmental toxin exposure directly causes endometriosis progression in humans are limited. Because women's health research has historically been underfunded, many important questions remain unanswered. Environmental toxins are therefore best understood as potential contributors to inflammatory burden rather than a single proven cause of disease.

Synthetic Fragrances

In perfumes, scented candles, detergents, air fresheners, and "fresh-smelling" cleaning products. These mixtures often contain phthalates and volatile organic compounds (VOCs) that bypass normal hormone signaling pathways.

Research: Exposure increases inflammatory reactivity and can aggravate hormone-sensitive conditions. *(Steinemann et al., Air Quality, Atmosphere & Health, 2016)*

Microplastics

Present in bottled water, food packaging, synthetic clothing fibers, cosmetics, cleaning products, and airborne dust released from household plastics. These tiny particles can enter the body through water, food, and inhalation. Once absorbed into the bloodstream, they are extremely difficult to eliminate because the body has no biological mechanism to break them down.

Research: Microplastics trigger oxidative stress, activate inflammatory pathways, and disrupt gut microbial balance — effects especially concerning for women with chronic inflammatory conditions. Long-term exposure has been linked to immune dysregulation and hormonal interference. *(Leslie et al., Environment International, 2022)*

Common Sources of Endocrine Disruptors in Daily Life

- plastic water bottles and food containers
- cosmetics, skincare, shampoos, deodorants
- household cleaning products
- perfumes, candles, air fresheners
- nonstick cookware
- contaminated tap water
- new furniture, mattresses, electronics
- packaged and ultra-processed foods

- pesticides on produce
- fast-food wrappers and takeout packaging

Most women are not simply reacting to "foods." They are reacting to cumulative inflammatory load — much of it coming from environmental toxins. Healing means lowering that load.

Bioaccumulation: Why These Chemicals Matter More for Women

Many endocrine disruptors are lipophilic, meaning they store in body fat — and women naturally have more body fat than men. Some EDCs also concentrate in:

- ovarian tissue
- breast tissue
- the endometrium
- the thyroid gland

This is one reason women experience higher rates of:

- endometriosis
- PCOS
- autoimmune disorders
- thyroid disease
- migraines
- unexplained infertility
- hormone-related cancers

Reducing chemical exposure is not optional for hormonal health — it is a powerful and essential part of lowering inflammation.

You're Not Meant to Live in Fear – You're Meant to Live Informed

Eliminating these triggers does not mean living in anxiety or obsessing over every product. It means:

- understanding what affects your body
- choosing safer alternatives at your own pace
- allowing your hormones and immune system to stabilize
- creating a home that supports your healing

Small changes compound. Just as toxins accumulate, so does wellness.

You have the power to build an environment that supports your body instead of inflaming it.

CHAPTER 7

FOODS THAT FUEL INFLAMMATION

Chronic inflammation doesn't begin with one dramatic trigger — it builds quietly, meal by meal, habit by habit. The foods we eat each day shape our hormones, digestion, microbiome, energy, and mood. Some foods nourish healing; others feed inflammation, increase oxidative stress, and overwhelm the immune system.

For women with endometriosis, PCOS, IBS, autoimmune tendencies, hormonal imbalance, or chronic fatigue, removing inflammatory foods is not a trend — it's a key part of healing. The intention is not to restrict you, but to reduce the burden on your system so your body finally has the capacity to rebalance and repair.

Below are foods scientifically shown to fuel inflammation — and why reducing or removing them can change everything.

1. Gluten – A Hidden Driver of Gut Inflammation

Gluten is a group of proteins found in wheat, rye, and barley. Even in people without celiac disease, gluten can increase intestinal permeability — the "leaky gut" effect — by triggering the release of zonulin, a protein that opens the tight junctions in the gut lining (Fasano, 2012).

A more permeable gut means:

- increased inflammation
- higher histamine reactivity
- immune activation
- worsened hormonal symptoms

For women with chronic illness, this is a major issue. Increased permeability allows bacterial fragments, toxins, and undigested food particles to enter the bloodstream, provoking an immune response that keeps the inflammatory cycle active.

Gluten also contains gluteomorphins — opioid-like peptides that can worsen cravings, bloating, and sluggish digestion.

You do not need celiac disease to be sensitive to gluten. Some individuals with conditions such as endometriosis, PCOS, thyroid disorders, IBS, or histamine intolerance report improvements when reducing or eliminating gluten as part of an anti-inflammatory diet.

Eliminating gluten today is far easier than it once was. There are countless gluten-free options that make the transition smooth and satisfying — including breads, pasta, pizza crusts, oatmeal, crackers, waffles, and wraps. Most grocery stores offer entire gluten-free sections, and many restaurants now provide gluten-free swaps without sacrificing flavor.

Removing gluten doesn't mean limiting variety — it's simply choosing different ingredients. Many options are even more nutrient-dense, especially when they're made from whole foods rather than refined flours. For example, pasta made from chickpeas, lentils, or quinoa offers higher protein and fiber. Pizza crusts can be made from cauliflower, almond flour, chickpeas, or rice flour. These alternatives support gut health, provide steady energy, and keep meals satisfying without triggering inflammation.

Gluten-free eating isn't restrictive when you choose foods that nourish you. It's just a different kind of abundance.

2. Dairy – Inflammatory, Hormone-Disrupting, and Often Misunderstood

Dairy is one of the most common triggers of inflammation, digestive distress, and hormonal imbalance — especially in women.

Why dairy can fuel inflammation:

- It often contains A1 casein, which breaks down into BCM-7, an inflammatory peptide linked to immune activation (Barnett et al., 2015).
- It is naturally high in histamine and can worsen IBS and endometriosis symptoms (Maintz & Novak, 2007).
- It raises IGF-1, a hormone associated with inflammation and acne (Melnik, 2011).
- Up to 70–75% of adults are lactose intolerant (Storhaug et al., 2017), which can cause bloating, gas, and fatigue.

Many women report significant improvements in cramps, bloating, energy, skin clarity, and PMS within weeks of removing dairy.

The ethical side of dairy

Even "ethical," "humane," or "organic" dairy production usually relies on separating newborn calves from their mothers so milk can be redirected to humans. Cows are repeatedly impregnated to maintain milk supply, and both mother and calf may experience distress. Many reports and investigations show that the term *"ethical"* often does not reflect a fundamentally different process — the same cycle of forced breeding, separation, and production remains. In other words, these labels improve marketing, but they rarely remove the practices themselves.

Removing dairy becomes both a health decision and a compassionate choice. You are free to move at your own pace, but it is worth knowing that reducing or eliminating dairy often supports both your body and your values.

3. Industrial Seed Oils – Silent Drivers of Inflammation

Seed oils — canola, soy, corn, sunflower, safflower, grapeseed, generic "vegetable oil" — are marketed as heart-healthy, yet research consistently links them to inflammation.

Why they inflame the body:

- They are extremely high in omega-6 linoleic acid, which converts into arachidonic acid, a precursor to inflammatory molecules (Johnson & Fritsche, 2012).
- They are often produced using high heat and chemical solvents like hexane, generating inflammatory oxidation byproducts.
- They disrupt the omega-6 : omega-3 balance, contributing to hormonal instability and immune dysregulation.

For women with chronic illness, seed oils can worsen:

- bloating
- cramps
- anxiety
- skin flares
- fatigue

Whenever possible, choose more stable, anti-inflammatory fats: extra-virgin olive oil, avocado oil, coconut oil, and naturally occurring fats from whole foods.

4. Highly Processed Foods – Manufactured Inflammation

Ultra-processed foods — packaged snacks, bars, flavored yogurts, frozen meals, many “diet” products, and even some “healthy” convenience items — burden the gut, liver, hormones, and immune system. Diets high in ultra-processed foods significantly increase inflammatory markers like CRP and IL-6 (Srour et al., 2019).

These foods are engineered to be hyper-palatable, shelf-stable, and addictive — not nourishing.

Modern marketing has made food labels difficult to trust. Words like “fit,” “bio,” “natural,” “healthy,” “high protein,” “low sugar,” or “clean” are often used as branding strategies to make highly processed products appear harmless.

Many snacks that look healthy still:

- contain emulsifiers
- use artificial sweeteners
- rely on cheap seed oils
- include multiple additives
- hide sugar under different names

What you can trust most is your own informed judgment.

A simple rule: **the fewer ingredients on the label, the better.** If a product contains ingredients you cannot pronounce, do not recognize, or cannot imagine growing in nature, your body will likely struggle to recognize them as food.

Common additives that may be problematic:

- Carboxymethylcellulose (CMC) – an emulsifier linked to gut permeability and dysbiosis (Chassaing et al., 2015)
- Polysorbate 80 – disrupts the gut lining and increases inflammation
- Maltodextrin – rapidly spikes blood sugar and feeds harmful bacteria
- High-fructose corn syrup (HFCS) – strongly pro-inflammatory
- Aspartame, sucralose, acesulfame potassium (Ace-K) – artificial sweeteners that alter microbiome composition
- Sodium benzoate – a preservative that can form benzene (a carcinogen) when combined with vitamin C
- BHA / BHT – synthetic antioxidants linked to endocrine disruption
- Monosodium glutamate (MSG) – flavor enhancer that can overstimulate neurotransmitters in sensitive individuals
- Carrageenan – a thickener associated with gut irritation and inflammation
- Propylene glycol – found in frostings, sauces, and flavored drinks
- "Natural flavors" – an umbrella term that can hide many compounds
- Industrial citric acid – often derived from mold and irritating for some sensitive guts

These ingredients do not nourish the body — they confuse it, burden it, and prolong inflammation.

If the ingredient list is long, scientific-sounding, or packed with additives, it is manufactured food, not nourishment. Slow, gentle healing begins by reducing foods that constantly activate the immune system and replacing them with foods your body recognizes.

5. Refined Sugar – Fuel for Inflammation, Hormonal Chaos, and Insulin Resistance

Sugar isn't just "empty calories." It drives inflammation through multiple pathways and places a heavy burden on the gut, hormones, liver, and nervous system.

Refined sugars:

- spike blood sugar, raising insulin and inflammatory cytokines
- feed harmful bacteria and Candida
- disrupt estrogen metabolism
- deplete magnesium and zinc (key nutrients for hormone balance)
- increase oxidative stress (Tappy, 2010)

For women with chronic illness, high sugar intake often worsens:

- PMS and cramps
- acne and breakouts
- mood swings
- fatigue
- bloating
- endometriosis pain
- anxiety
- sleep disruption

But sugar is only part of the picture.

Artificial Sweeteners – "Sugar-Free" but Often More Disruptive

Many women reach for "diet," "zero," or "sugar-free" products believing they are better options. Yet artificial sweeteners can be even more disruptive than sugar for some people.

Common artificial sweeteners include:

- aspartame
- sucralose (Splenda)
- acesulfame-K (Ace-K)
- saccharin
- neotame
- advantame

Research shows these compounds can:

- disrupt the gut microbiome and reduce beneficial bacteria (Suez et al., 2014)
- trigger glucose intolerance
- increase cravings
- interfere with appetite regulation
- worsen anxiety and mood instability

They provide sweetness without calories, but they confuse the body's metabolic signaling.

Diet Soda – One of the Most Metabolically Damaging Choices

Diet soda is often marketed as a healthy alternative, yet studies suggest the opposite. Even without sugar, diet soda can:

- increase insulin resistance (Romero et al., 2016)

- raise the risk of metabolic syndrome
- alter gut microbiome composition
- increase abdominal fat
- destabilize blood sugar
- worsen inflammation

The sweet taste alone can trigger an insulin response: the body prepares for sugar and receives chemicals instead.

Diet sodas also typically contain:

- artificial sweeteners (aspartame, sucralose)
- caramel coloring
- phosphoric acid
- sodium benzoate
- "natural flavors"

For women with endometriosis, PCOS, thyroid disorders, or IBS, diet soda is a common but overlooked trigger for flares, bloating, and fatigue.

What About Monk Fruit and Stevia?

Not all sugar substitutes are equally problematic. Pure monk fruit extract and pure stevia extract can be reasonable options for many people, especially in small amounts. The issue is that most commercial products are blends that include:

- erythritol
- maltodextrin
- dextrose
- inulin
- flavorings

These blends behave more like ultra-processed additives and can irritate the gut.

Safer options include:

- pure monk fruit extract (without fillers)
- pure stevia extract (if tolerated)
- whole fruit
- small amounts of raw honey or dates
- spices like cinnamon, vanilla, and cacao for natural sweetness

If an alternative has multiple ingredients or anything you cannot identify, it's best to be cautious.

A Healthier Relationship With Sweetness

You do not need to eliminate sweetness — you are simply returning it to sources your body understands. When sweetness comes from whole foods and minimal, clean ingredients, it is less likely to fuel inflammation and more likely to support hormonal and emotional balance.

The Sugar Detox Effect – Why Cravings Disappear

Sugar can be habit-forming. The dopamine surge from sweet foods conditions the brain to want more, and the crash that follows keeps the cycle going.

But after even about seven days of significantly reducing sugar, many people notice:

- fewer cravings
- more stable energy
- calmer mood

- less bloating
- improved sleep

The first days can be uncomfortable, but the freedom that follows is often profound. For many women, reducing sugar becomes one of the most transformative steps for long-term health.

CHAPTER 8

THE TRUTH ABOUT ALCOHOL AND INFLAMMATION

Alcohol is one of the most overlooked drivers of inflammation — especially for women with endometriosis, PCOS, IBS, thyroid disorders, autoimmune tendencies, anxiety, or chronic fatigue. Even small amounts can disrupt hormones, irritate the gut lining, tax the liver, and destabilize the nervous system.

Many women do everything "right" — they clean up their diet, take supplements, and reduce stress — yet continue to struggle with bloating, anxiety, mood swings, fatigue, sleep disturbances, or painful flares. Often, alcohol is the missing link.

What makes alcohol particularly harmful is not just the drink itself, but the entire biological chain reaction it triggers:

- inflammation
- hormonal imbalance
- gut irritation
- histamine overload
- neurotransmitter disruption

- sleep disturbance
- blood-sugar instability

For women with chronic illness, alcohol is rarely neutral. It is a biological stressor that can fuel the very symptoms you are working so hard to heal. Understanding how alcohol affects your body is one of the most powerful actions you can take toward long-term relief.

1. The Hidden Mechanism Behind Alcohol's "Relaxation"

Alcohol acts on the brain's GABA and dopamine systems — the same neurotransmitters involved in calm and pleasure. This is why a drink may initially feel warm, social, or relaxing.

But this calm is temporary and chemically driven.

As soon as the body begins metabolizing alcohol, the brain rebounds in the opposite direction.

Levels of:

- glutamate (an excitatory neurotransmitter)
- cortisol (a stress hormone)
- adrenaline

all rise.

This rebound can cause:

- anxiety
- irritability
- racing thoughts
- restlessness
- elevated heart rate
- "hangxiety"

- shallow or disrupted sleep

What feels soothing in the moment often becomes internal agitation hours later. This is not a character flaw — it is physiology.

2. Why Alcohol Affects Women More Strongly

Women metabolize alcohol differently than men, and this difference is especially important for those with chronic inflammation.

Women typically have:

- lower levels of alcohol dehydrogenase (ADH), the enzyme that breaks down alcohol
- a higher percentage of body fat, which keeps alcohol more concentrated
- hormonal fluctuations, particularly estrogen, that intensify alcohol's effects
- slower clearance of toxic acetaldehyde

This means that the same amount of alcohol can result in:

- higher blood alcohol levels
- deeper liver stress
- stronger inflammatory responses
- more intense hormonal disruption
- greater anxiety afterwards
- more PMS and cycle-related symptoms

Research shows that women experience more pronounced alcohol-induced liver stress, hormonal shifts, and inflammation than men (Erol & Karpyak, 2015). For women with endometriosis, PCOS, IBS, or autoimmune tendencies, this impact is even more relevant.

3. How Alcohol Triggers Inflammation

Alcohol affects multiple organs and systems in a cascade.

Step 1 — The liver enters emergency mode
The liver converts alcohol into acetaldehyde, a compound up to 30 times more toxic than ethanol (Seitz & Stickel, 2007). During this detox process, the liver temporarily deprioritizes:

- hormone metabolism
- blood sugar regulation
- environmental detoxification
- histamine breakdown

Inflammatory cytokines increase, signaling the immune system that something is wrong.

Step 2 — Alcohol damages the gut lining ("leaky gut")
Alcohol can:

- erode the protective mucus layer in the gut
- widen tight junctions between intestinal cells
- increase intestinal permeability

This allows endotoxins to enter the bloodstream and trigger systemic inflammation (Bishehsari et al., 2017).

Common symptoms include:

- bloating
- heaviness
- digestive discomfort
- headaches
- brain fog
- skin irritation

- fatigue
- increased pain

Step 3 — Alcohol and histamine: a double hit

Alcohol is a strong histamine trigger. It:

1. **Releases histamine**
   Alcohol stimulates mast cells, which can cause flushing, headaches, itching, anxiety, congestion, or nausea.

2. **Blocks DAO (diamine oxidase)**
   DAO is the enzyme responsible for breaking down histamine in the gut. Alcohol suppresses DAO, allowing histamine to build up (Maintz & Novak, 2007).

3. **Increases intestinal permeability**
   A more permeable gut allows more histamine-producing bacteria and endotoxins to enter the bloodstream.

This combination makes alcohol one of the strongest everyday triggers for women with endometriosis, IBS, migraines, or histamine intolerance.

Step 4 — The hormonal ripple effect

Because the liver is busy processing alcohol, it becomes less efficient at clearing:

- estrogen
- cortisol
- histamine

This can lead to:

- estrogen dominance
- PMS and breast tenderness
- ovulation pain
- mood swings
- insomnia
- anxiety

Women with hormonal imbalance often feel the effects of a single drink for several days.

4. What Alcohol Does to Your Body in Six Hours

0–30 minutes: Dopamine & GABA rush
Sedation, warmth, and lowered inhibition. The liver shifts into emergency detox mode.

30–90 minutes: Acetaldehyde toxicity
Inflammation rises. Cytokines are released. The brain and liver experience increased stress.

90 minutes–3 hours: Blood sugar crash & gut disruption
Cortisol and adrenaline rise. The gut lining weakens. Blood sugar becomes unstable.

3–6 hours: Stress rebound
GABA drops. Glutamate surges. Nighttime anxiety and early awakenings often occur.

6+ hours: Lingering inflammation
Oxidative stress, inflammatory markers, and hormonal imbalance can persist for 24 hours or more.

This is why even one drink can cause bloating, anxiety, irritability, and fatigue the next day.

5. Alcohol and Sleep: How It Disrupts Your Nervous System

Alcohol induces sedation, not restorative sleep. It alters sleep architecture in several ways:

1. **Suppressed REM sleep**
   REM is crucial for emotional processing and nervous-system repair. Alcohol can reduce REM sleep by up to 40% (Roehrs & Roth, 2001).

2. **Invcreased nighttime awakenings**
   As alcohol wears off and glutamate rises, many people experience 2–4 AM wakeups with racing thoughts or sweating.

3. **Elevated cortisol and heart rate**
   Even a single drink can raise nighttime cortisol and keep heart rate elevated, preventing full rest.

4. **Reduced deep sleep**
   Deep, slow-wave sleep is where much of physical healing occurs — and alcohol significantly reduces time spent in this phase.

Poor sleep alone raises inflammation, worsens pain, and destabilizes hormones.

6. The Paradox: Why Alcohol Feels Good but Makes You Feel Worse

The dopamine boost from alcohol is brief. Once it fades, dopamine levels drop below baseline, which can lead to:

- low energy
- low mood

- emotional flatness
- anxiety

This is a mild form of biochemical withdrawal — even from moderate drinking.

At the same time, acetaldehyde depletes glutathione, one of the body's most important antioxidants for detoxification, inflammation control, and emotional stability (Wu et al., 2004). This contributes to:

- irritability
- brain fog
- inflammation
- heightened pain
- fatigue

Alcohol temporarily mimics joy while diminishing your body's natural ability to feel calm and well.

7. What Happens When You Stop or Reduce Alcohol

Within weeks of significantly reducing alcohol, the body begins to reset. Many women notice:

- stronger gut integrity
- better microbiome diversity
- more efficient liver function
- smoother estrogen clearance
- fewer histamine reactions
- more stable cortisol and mood
- deeper, more restorative sleep
- less pain and bloating
- brighter skin
- more stable energy

This is not coincidence — it is the body returning to balance.

8. Why Cravings Disappear When You Stop Drinking

As with sugar, something powerful happens when you stop drinking: the cravings often fade. Alcohol creates a sharp dopamine spike followed by a steep drop. That drop is what drives the urge for another drink.

Once you stop drinking for 7–14 days, many people experience:

- more stable dopamine levels
- lower cortisol
- improved sleep
- better blood-sugar control
- reduced anxiety
- a calmer nervous system

The craving disappears not because you became "stronger," but because the chemical imbalance that fueled it is no longer being constantly triggered.

What once felt like comfort loses its hold, and you begin to feel how good your body can truly be allowed to feel. Alcohol never created relaxation — it borrowed it from tomorrow. When you step away from it, you allow your body to experience real relaxation, clarity, and stability.

For years, some studies suggested that moderate alcohol intake — especially red wine — might offer cardiovascular benefits. However, more recent independent analyses have revealed that many of these associations were influenced by confounding lifestyle factors and, in some cases, by industry-funded research shaping how results were interpreted (Stockwell et al., 2016). Updated reviews now emphasize that there is no medical reason to start drinking alcohol for health purposes and that for most people, the risks outweigh any proposed benefits (GBD 2022 Alcohol Collaborators, 2022).

WHAT ABOUT RESVERATROL?

Red wine contains resveratrol, an antioxidant often promoted for heart health, but the levels in a typical glass are extremely small. Clinical trials showing benefits used doses far higher than those achievable through wine consumption (Novelle et al., 2015). More recent research confirms that meaningful therapeutic levels would require consuming unsafe amounts of alcohol (Galbete et al., 2023).

Fortunately, resveratrol and similar polyphenols occur abundantly in foods such as grapes, blueberries, cranberries, and peanuts — and these deliver antioxidant benefits without alcohol-induced inflammation, gut disruption, or hormonal imbalance (Chiva-Blanch & Visioli, 2012).

If you enjoy an occasional drink, that is a personal choice.
But it is important to be clear: **alcohol is not a health-promoting substance**, and the compounds once used to justify its "benefits" can be obtained far more safely from whole plant foods.

PART III

FOOD, GUT & TOOLS FOR DAILY REGULATION

CHAPTER 9

CYCLE-SYNCED EATING

Women do not run on a fixed, unchanging biological schedule. While men follow a relatively stable 24-hour hormonal rhythm, a woman's hormones shift throughout a four-phase monthly cycle. These shifts influence digestion, metabolism, inflammation sensitivity, cravings, mood, energy, and stress resilience.

Most women are taught to expect sameness: same productivity, same appetite, same workouts, same emotional stability every day. When our biology naturally adjusts, many of us try to override it — pushing through fatigue, restricting food when metabolism increases, or forcing intense exercise when hormones make the body more vulnerable to inflammation.

Cycle-synced eating is not about controlling the body or following strict rules. It is about working *with* your biology instead of against it. When you understand what your body needs at each phase, food becomes permission, not restriction. Supporting the cycle reduces inflammation, stabilizes hormones, and makes the entire month feel steadier and more predictable.

Each of the four phases below includes **optimal foods, recommended movement, and emotional support** to help your body do what it is designed to do: repair, ovulate, detoxify, and rebalance.

MENSTRUAL PHASE (DAYS 1–5)

Low hormones · Lower energy · Higher inflammation sensitivity

During menstruation, estrogen and progesterone reach their lowest levels. The body redirects resources toward shedding and rebuilding the uterine lining, which is why many women experience increased fatigue, slower digestion, heightened emotional sensitivity, and sometimes intensified pain responses. This phase requires warmth, nourishment, and rest to minimize inflammatory stress.

Optimal Foods

Focus on warm, mineral-rich meals that replenish nutrients and reduce prostaglandin-related pain:

- cooked leafy greens, lentils, beans, pumpkin seeds, quinoa, and other iron-rich foods
- soups, stews, broths, porridges, slow-cooked vegetables, braised root vegetables
- magnesium-rich foods such as avocado, cacao, chia seeds, tahini, and leafy greens
- anti-inflammatory fats such as olive oil, flaxseed, hemp, and fatty plant-based sources
- warming herbs such as ginger, cinnamon, turmeric, fennel, cumin, and cardamom

Cold foods are not "forbidden," but warm meals are easier to digest while the body directs energy toward uterine repair. This phase is not the ideal time to experiment with new foods. Because the body is busy shedding the uterine lining, digestion can be more sensitive. Warm, familiar, easy-to-digest meals help reduce cramps, stabilize blood sugar, and support mineral replenishment. New foods are easier to introduce later in the cycle, when digestion and inflammation are more stable.

Movement

Choose circulation-supportive activity that does not elevate cortisol or exhaust the nervous system. Ideal options include:

- slow walking
- gentle Pilates or stretching
- restorative or yin-style yoga
- mobility work or light fascia release

This is not a time to "push through." Resting builds resilience; overexertion increases inflammation.

Emotional & Nervous System Support

Lower estrogen means lower serotonin activity, which can heighten stress reactivity. Treat emotional sensitivity as physiology, not a flaw. Support this phase by:

- protecting quiet time or privacy when possible
- avoiding heavy planning or conflict when feasible
- choosing warmth (heat pads, baths, herbal teas)
- limiting caffeine if it worsens cramps or anxiety

Respecting your body's slower pace during menstruation reduces systemic inflammation and sets the stage for a calmer cycle.

FOLLICULAR PHASE (DAYS 6–13)

Rising estrogen · Rising energy · Improved digestion and metabolism

As menstruation ends, estrogen rises. The body becomes more insulin-sensitive, digestion improves, mood lifts, and the nervous system becomes more resilient to stress. This is a phase of renewal — the body prepares for ovulation, making it an ideal time to introduce variety, fiber, and lighter meals that support microbiome balance.

Optimal Foods

Emphasize fresh, fiber-rich foods that support healthy estrogen metabolism and gut microbial diversity:

- colorful vegetables and salads (tolerated better during this phase)
- cruciferous vegetables such as broccoli, cauliflower, cabbage, and arugula
- sprouted legumes, chickpeas, hummus, beans, lentils
- seeds, berries, citrus fruits, and lightly steamed greens
- probiotic foods like sauerkraut, kimchi, coconut yogurt, or miso (if well tolerated)

Because digestion is generally more efficient and blood sugar more stable during the follicular phase, this can be a supportive time to try new foods or recipes — especially if you're expanding plant-based meals.

Movement

With rising estrogen, the body recovers faster and tolerates more exertion. Support this window with strength-building activity:

- strength training or resistance workouts
- cycling, jogging, swimming, moderate cardio
- Pilates or barre with progressive load

This is also the best time to challenge the body — not with intensity for punishment, but with movement that builds strength for the rest of the month.

Emotional & Nervous System Support

This phase brings clearer thinking, openness, and enthusiasm. Use this energy thoughtfully:

- initiate new habits or projects
- plan social activities or tasks requiring creativity
- set goals or organize schedules

The follicular phase is biologically aligned with expansion. Let energy rise without rushing or burning it out.

OVULATORY PHASE (DAYS 14–17)

Peak estrogen · Increased inflammation sensitivity · Higher sociability and libido

Ovulation is the most hormonal event of the month. Estrogen peaks, a small surge of testosterone boosts confidence and libido, and the body becomes slightly warmer. Digestion may speed up, and many women feel more extroverted, articulate, and energetic. However, inflammation can spike if the body is stressed or deprived.

Optimal Foods

Support liver detoxification, antioxidant balance, and bowel regularity to help metabolize excess estrogen:

- berries, cherries, pomegranate, citrus fruits
- cruciferous vegetables (broccoli, cabbage, watercress)
- zucchini, bell peppers, leafy greens, fresh herbs
- flaxseed and chia (supporting estrogen elimination)
- antioxidant-rich spices (turmeric, garlic, oregano, basil)

Raw foods are generally tolerated best here, but they are not required. Prioritize antioxidants and fiber.

Movement

Energy is often at its peak. Choose workouts that combine strength, endurance, and dynamic movement:

- HIIT or interval training (only if well-recovered)
- power or tempo-focused strength training
- dance, cycling, running, or athletic conditioning

If you feel more energetic, lean into it — but do not force intensity. Pain or fatigue means inflammation is already elevated.

Emotional & Nervous System Support

This phase favors communication, confidence, and collaboration. It can also increase emotional intensity if personal needs are being ignored. Support yourself by:

- expressing needs clearly
- using this window for relationship discussions, presentations, planning
- avoiding overcommitment or oversocializing

Your body is primed for connection and productivity — honor it without overwhelming it.

LUTEAL PHASE (DAYS 18–28)

Rising progesterone · Higher cravings · Lower stress tolerance

After ovulation, progesterone rises. Metabolic rate increases — meaning many women genuinely need more calories during this phase. Digestion slows slightly, blood sugar becomes less stable, and serotonin levels fluctuate, which is why cravings, mood changes, anxiety, or bloating may appear, especially if the body is under-supported.

This is not a lack of willpower. It is biology shifting into preparation and protection.

Optimal Foods

Support blood sugar stability, reduce inflammation, and ease progesterone-related digestive slowdowns:

- starchy vegetables (sweet potatoes, squash, beets, carrots)
- complex carbohydrates (quinoa, oats, gluten-free whole grains)
- fiber-rich vegetables (cooked greens, artichoke, Brussels sprouts)
- magnesium- and B-vitamin-rich foods (nuts, seeds, legumes)
- warming herbs and broths to support digestion

Increasing complex carbs prevents cravings and binge-restrict cycles. Restricting food triggers cortisol, blood sugar crashes, and irritability during this phase.

Movement

Focus on slow-burn strength and restorative rhythm:

- moderate strength training
- Pilates or controlled movement exercises
- low-impact cardio
- stretching, light yoga, fascia and lymph work

Support circulation without overloading the nervous system.

Emotional & Nervous System Support

Progesterone increases sensitivity to stress; dopamine and serotonin fluctuate. Support yourself by:

- prioritizing sleep, slower evenings, and warm meals
- reducing caffeine, alcohol, and sugar (they worsen PMS, acne, and anxiety)
- creating boundaries around social or emotional drain
- preparing ahead with nourishing meals to avoid reactive eating

Your body is asking for steadiness and predictability — not intensity or perfection.

Optional Support: Seed Cycling

Seed cycling is a gentle, food-based ritual some women use to support hormonal balance across the month. It is not a magic cure or a replacement for medical care, and research is still emerging. But many women find that it helps regulate cycles, ease PMS, and support skin and mood — and it fits beautifully within an anti-inflammatory, plant-rich way of eating.

The idea is simple: you rotate specific seeds through the menstrual cycle to provide targeted nutrients and fatty acids that may support estrogen and progesterone balance.

- **Follicular phase (Days 1–14)**
  Focus on seeds that support healthy estrogen metabolism:
  – **Ground flaxseed** – provides lignans that help modulate estrogen and support detoxification in the liver and gut.
  – **Pumpkin seeds** – rich in zinc, which supports ovarian function, immune balance, and early-cycle hormone production.
  Aim for **1–2 tablespoons of ground flaxseed + 1–2 tablespoons of pumpkin seeds per day**, added to smoothies, chia pudding, salads, soups, or gluten-free oatmeal.

- **Luteal phase (Days 15–28)**
  Shift toward seeds that support progesterone, nervous system calm, and mineral balance:
  – **Sesame seeds** – provide lignans and minerals (especially calcium and magnesium) that support hormone metabolism and stress resilience.
  – **Sunflower seeds** – rich in vitamin E and selenium, which support progesterone production, thyroid health, and antioxidant defense.
  Again, aim for **1–2 tablespoons of sesame seeds + 1–2 tablespoons of sunflower seeds per day**, sprinkled over meals or blended into sauces and dressings (tahini, seed butters, seed-based dips).

You do not need exact timing for this to be helpful. If your cycle is irregular or you are on hormonal birth control, you can still use seed cycling by following a **simple two-week rhythm**:

- Days 1–14 of any month: flax + pumpkin
- Days 15–28 of any month: sesame + sunflower

This gives your body consistent access to the nutrients involved in hormone metabolism, regardless of exact cycle length.

Seed cycling is not about perfection or strict rules. Think of it as a nourishing ritual — a small daily act that supports your cycle, your gut, and your nervous system at the same time. Even if the hormonal effects are subtle, the benefits of fiber, minerals, and healthy fats are very real. Over time, many women notice that adding these seeds contributes to:

- more stable energy and mood,
- gentler PMS,
- better bowel regularity,
- and feeling more grounded in their bodies throughout the month.

Like everything in this book, seed cycling is an invitation, not an obligation. If it feels supportive, keep it. If it feels overwhelming, you can set it aside and still experience deep healing through the other foundations of your Reset.

CYCLE-SYNCING AS A FORM OF SELF-REGULATION

Working with your cycle teaches you to listen rather than control. Each phase requires something different — warmth, lightness, antioxidants, or stability — not to restrict you, but to support what your body is already doing. When you stop expecting sameness and start feeding your biology as it changes, inflammation eases, cravings calm, periods become lighter, and emotional regulation improves.

Cycle-synced eating is not a trend; it's a return to partnership with your physiology. But like any partnership, it's personal. This framework provides a foundation, yet each woman's experience is unique — especially for those with endometriosis, PCOS, IBS, or who are on hormonal birth control.

For example, many guides describe ovulation as a "high-energy" phase, but for me it has often been the most draining part of the cycle. My pain and fatigue peak when estrogen peaks, which taught me that my body needs extra support for estrogen metabolism during this phase. I know women who experience the opposite — they feel strong during ovulation and require more support during menstruation or luteal days. The point isn't to force yourself into a model; it's to use the model as a starting point and let your own body show you the specifics.

Cycle-syncing gives the map. Your body teaches the details.

CHAPTER 10

MACRONUTRIENT HARMONY: HOW THE THREE WORK TOGETHER

Macronutrient harmony is not a diet strategy — it is the foundation of metabolic, hormonal, and inflammatory balance.

Women's bodies work through constant biochemical communication. Proteins, fats, and carbohydrates are not independent nutrients competing for space on a plate — they are a cooperative triad influencing mood, hormones, cellular repair, immune signaling, microbiome balance, and energy stability. When these nutrients arrive in balanced proportions, the body feels supported instead of threatened. Blood sugar stabilizes, cravings diminish, inflammation decreases, and the nervous system becomes calmer.

In contrast, when one macronutrient is missing or consistently overconsumed — such as an excess of refined carbohydrates or a lack of healthy fats — the body responds with instability: mood swings, bloating, cravings, fatigue, inflammation, or disrupted sleep. Hormones and neurotransmitters cannot regulate properly when the body is undernourished or imbalanced. For women, whose endocrine systems respond quickly to stress, digestion, and glucose fluctuations, balanced meals create internal stability that supports healing.

Balanced nutrition is not restrictive. It is how the body maintains homeostasis — a state where inflammation can settle, metabolism can function, and hormones can regulate without constantly compensating for imbalance

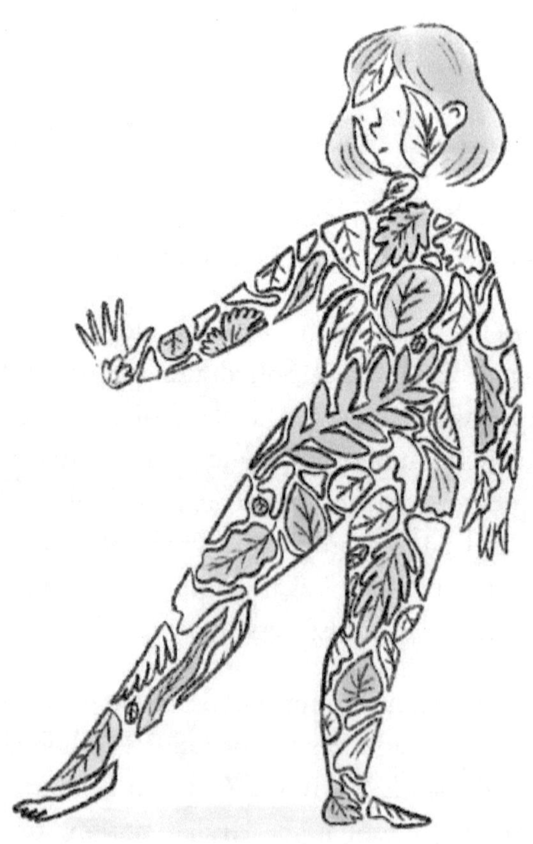

WHY MACRONUTRIENT BALANCE IS THE FOUNDATION OF HEALING

Macronutrient balance supports the body as a unified system, not isolated parts. When meals include fiber-rich carbohydrates, healthy fats, and meaningful protein, the body experiences a steady influx of glucose, satiety signals, and anti-inflammatory nutrients. This combination prevents cortisol spikes, supports insulin sensitivity, and builds a predictable energy rhythm throughout the day.

Women, in particular, feel the effects of imbalance more strongly due to the interaction between blood sugar and sex hormones. Cycling hormones influence appetite, metabolism, and neurotransmitters. A meal that is balanced provides emotional steadiness, better PMS symptoms, and lower inflammatory responses throughout the cycle.

A healing body does not require extremes — only consistency.

CARBOHYDRATES: ENERGY, SEROTONIN, AND STEADY MOOD

Carbohydrates are the brain's preferred fuel. Too little carbohydrate intake can trigger irritability, fatigue, sleep disruption, and intense cravings because carbohydrates influence serotonin production — the neurotransmitter responsible for emotional stability, appetite regulation, and restful sleep.

Popular low-carbohydrate diets can be particularly destabilizing for women. Female physiology is sensitive to drops in glucose, especially during menstruation and the luteal phase. When carbohydrates are too restricted, cortisol rises, hunger increases, sleep worsens, and emotional volatility becomes more likely.

However, not all carbohydrates behave the same way. Refined carbohydrates — pastries, white bread, sugary snacks, sweetened drinks — cause sharp blood sugar spikes followed by steep crashes, triggering cortisol, cravings, and anxiety. In contrast, slow-digesting carbohydrates from whole plant foods deliver gradual, steady energy because they come packaged with fiber and minerals. Examples include sweet potatoes, lentils, chickpeas, beans, oats, quinoa, vegetables, and berries. These foods stabilize blood sugar, reduce inflammation, and provide emotional steadiness throughout the day.

THE ROLE OF FIBER

Fiber is one of the most undervalued components of an anti-inflammatory diet. It supports the microbiome, helps the body eliminate excess hormones and inflammatory byproducts, regulates bowel movements, and keeps blood sugar stable. Research from the Harvard T.H. Chan School of Public Health shows that adequate fiber intake lowers systemic inflammation and improves estrogen metabolism — both essential in conditions like endometriosis, PCOS, and IBS (Harvard T.H. Chan School of Public Health, 2020).

There are two main types of fiber that work together in the body:

- **Soluble fiber** (found in chia seeds, oats, beans, lentils, and some fruits) forms a gel-like consistency during digestion. This slows down the absorption of glucose, prevents spikes and crashes in energy, and feeds beneficial gut bacteria.

- **Insoluble fiber** (found in vegetables, seeds, and certain whole grains) adds bulk to the stool and speeds up transit time. This is crucial because excess estrogen and inflammatory compounds are cleared through the bowel

— when elimination is slow, they can be reabsorbed and worsen symptoms.

Consistent intake of both types supports hormonal stability, smoother digestion, better bowel regularity, reduced bloating, and more steady energy. Most women feel best with 25–35 grams of fiber per day, increasing gradually and pairing it with adequate hydration to prevent gas or discomfort.

Supporting fiber doesn't mean adding high-fiber products — it means prioritizing real, diverse whole foods that nourish the gut and help the body clear what it no longer needs.

HEALTHY FATS: THE ARCHITECTURE OF HORMONES AND CELLULAR HEALTH

Healthy fats are structural material for hormones. Estrogen, progesterone, cortisol, and thyroid hormones require fat to be produced and transported. Brain tissue, cell membranes, and immune cells also depend on fatty acids for communication, repair, and anti-inflammatory activity.

The issue is not fat itself but the type consumed. Modern diets contain an excess of omega-6 fats from industrial seed oils (corn, soybean, sunflower, safflower, canola). These oils increase the production of prostaglandin E2 (PGE2), associated with menstrual cramps, pelvic pain, and chronic inflammatory activation. Elevated PGE2 is documented in endometriosis and other inflammatory conditions (Bulun, 2019).

Conversely, omega-3 fats (from flax, chia, hemp, walnuts, and algae oil) help produce prostaglandin E3 (PGE3), which reduces inflammation and softens pain responses. Omega-3s also support the production of resolvins and protectins — specialized molecules that actively help the immune system shut off inflammation when it is no longer needed (Serhan, 2014).

Research shows omega-3 intake is associated with reduced menstrual pain, improved immune regulation, and lower inflammatory responses in pelvic disorders (Harel, 1996; Rahbar et al., 2012). Women often notice calmer cycles, less bloating, and more stable mood when omega-3 intake becomes consistent.

Plant-based omega-3 sources

- Ground flaxseed (ALA + lignans for estrogen metabolism)
- Chia seeds (soothing gel for gut lining + glucose stability)
- Hemp seeds (complete protein + balanced fatty acids)
- Walnuts (polyphenols + cardiovascular support)
- Algae oil (direct EPA/DHA alternative to fish oil)

Healthy fats help regulate hormones, appetite, emotional resilience, and tissue repair — especially when paired with balanced carbohydrates and protein.

PROTEIN: REPAIR, HORMONAL STABILITY, AND CELLULAR RENEWAL

Protein is often misunderstood as a nutrient only for building muscle, yet it plays a central role in healing. Proteins break down into amino acids that repair the gut lining, immune cells, connective tissue, enzymes, and neurotransmitters. Without adequate protein, the body prioritizes survival over repair, slowing healing and destabilizing hormones. Low intake can contribute to fatigue, low immunity, brittle hair or nails, slower digestion, and difficulty managing cravings due to unstable blood glucose. Amino acids also support liver detoxification, which is essential for clearing used hormones, inflammatory molecules, and environmental toxins.

Plant-based proteins — lentils, chickpeas, tofu, tempeh, quinoa, hemp seeds, chia, green peas, and spirulina — provide anti-inflammatory advantages and offer fiber, unlike many animal proteins. Women generally benefit from simply including a meaningful protein source at each meal rather than obsessively tracking grams. Most women feel best aiming for around 1.0–1.2 g of protein per kilogram of body weight per day, or slightly more when healing, training, or living with chronic conditions (Rodriguez et al., 2009; Phillips & Van Loon, 2011).

Starting the day with protein makes a measurable difference. A protein-rich breakfast supports appetite regulation, cognitive clarity, and stable energy throughout the day (UCLA Oppenheimer Center for Neurobiology of Stress & Resilience, 2024). Higher breakfast protein intake has also been associated with improvements in lean body mass and skeletal muscle index (Schulenburg et al., 2023). Research highlights that women who consume protein earlier in the day experience fewer cravings and better hormonal balance due to steadier blood sugar and reduced cortisol spikes (Blue Cross Blue Shield of Michigan, 2022).

Plant-based protein breakfast ideas

- Chia pudding made with fortified almond or soy milk, topped with berries and pumpkin seeds
- Tofu scramble seasoned with turmeric and black salt, served with sautéed spinach or mushrooms
- Overnight oats with hemp seeds, ground flaxseed, almond butter, and cinnamon
- Protein smoothie (soy milk or pea-protein base) with blueberries, spinach, chia, and cacao
- Quinoa breakfast bowl with warm coconut milk, cinnamon, tahini, and sliced banana

- Chickpea flour pancakes (besan) with fruit compote or date-sweetened tahini drizzle

Including protein with breakfast slows carbohydrate absorption, which prevents sharp glucose spikes and cortisol surges that often lead to cravings, irritability, or mid-morning fatigue. Paired with healthy fats and fiber, protein helps maintain steadier appetite cues, clearer thinking, and calmer energy — creating a foundation for hormonal balance throughout the day.

THE HEALING PLATE FRAMEWORK

A healing diet is not about measuring portions or counting calories — it is about consistency and construction. A balanced plate supports digestion, hormonal regulation, and metabolic health by combining:

- fiber-rich vegetables
- slow-digesting carbohydrates
- meaningful protein
- healthy fats to improve absorption

When these components coexist, glucose stabilizes, inflammatory pathways calm, and energy becomes predictable. Digestion improves because the body is not overwhelmed by one macronutrient in isolation. Hormones stabilize because cortisol, insulin, and reproductive hormones are regulated through consistent nutrient delivery.

This framework adapts to any cuisine or lifestyle. It is simple enough to maintain during busy weeks and powerful enough to support long-term healing.

WHAT BALANCED MEALS LOOK LIKE

To make this structure more tangible, here are several examples of balanced meals that follow the macronutrient harmony approach. These are not recipes — simply combinations that illustrate what a healing plate can look like.

- A grounding breakfast might be a chia–oat pudding made with plant milk, a scoop of protein powder, fresh berries, and a spoonful of ground flaxseed.
- Another option is a sweet potato bowl with coconut yogurt, walnuts, and cinnamon, offering slow carbohydrates, healthy fats, and natural fiber.
- A green smoothie with spinach, banana, hemp seeds, protein powder, and almond butter delivers a nutrient-dense, easily digestible morning meal.

Lunch can be built around vibrant plant combinations:

- A quinoa and chickpea salad with kale, avocado, and pumpkin seeds drizzled with olive oil provides lasting satiety and a broad spectrum of micronutrients.
- Lentil soup paired with steamed broccoli and brown rice offers warmth and stability.
- Tofu stir-fried with mixed vegetables and buckwheat noodles creates a balanced, energizing midday dish.

Dinner can be soothing and restorative:

- A baked sweet potato topped with black beans and tahini, served alongside sautéed greens, creates a deeply satisfying evening meal.

- A vegetable curry made with tofu, coconut milk, turmeric, and quinoa brings warmth and anti-inflammatory benefits.
- Roasted seasonal vegetables served with lentils and arugula lightly dressed with hemp oil provide nourishment without heaviness.

Snacks can be kept simple but strategic — coconut yogurt with chia, an apple paired with almond butter, or walnuts with a handful of berries all support blood sugar without overstimulation.

These examples show how easy it is to create balanced meals once you understand the principles. You do not need to obsess over exact macronutrient quantities; your body responds best when these elements appear naturally together.

COMMON EATING PATTERNS THAT DISRUPT BALANCE

Many women unintentionally weaken metabolic and hormonal balance through eating patterns shaped by stress, rushed schedules, emotional eating, or diet culture:

- Carbohydrates alone (fruit, toast, pastries, snacks without fat or protein) cause glucose spikes followed by crashes, leading to anxiety, cravings, and irritability.
- Skipping breakfast or replacing it with coffee raises cortisol, destabilizes blood sugar for the entire day, and worsens PMS.
- Fear of healthy fats — a legacy of outdated diet messaging — leads to deficient hormone production and emotional instability.
- Low-protein diets reduce tissue repair, impair detoxification, and exacerbate cravings and fatigue.

- Reliance on inflammatory seed oils found in packaged foods and restaurant meals increases prostaglandin activity linked to menstrual pain and pelvic inflammation.

Recognizing these patterns is not about guilt — it's about clarity. With awareness, change becomes intuitive rather than restrictive.

HOW MACRONUTRIENTS INFLUENCE MOOD, ANXIETY, AND SLEEP

Food is biochemical communication. Carbohydrates influence serotonin, healthy fats modulate neuroinflammation and cell communication, and proteins provide amino acids for dopamine, GABA, and serotonin synthesis. When meals are balanced, neurotransmitters stabilize, and emotional regulation becomes easier.

Unbalanced meals or skipped meals trigger cortisol spikes, leading to irritability, anxiety, and disrupted sleep. Chronically unstable blood sugar mirrors emotional instability. A balanced plate supports both physical healing and mental steadiness.

Women often notice less irritability, fewer cravings, deeper sleep, and calmer moods simply from eating balanced meals consistently.

MACRONUTRIENTS IN CHRONIC ILLNESS AND INFLAMMATION

For women with endometriosis, PCOS, autoimmune conditions, IBS, or chronic fatigue, macronutrient harmony reduces inflammatory load and supports metabolism, detoxification, and pain reduction.

- Stable glucose lowers cortisol and inflammatory cytokine release.

- Adequate protein supports glutathione production, the body's master antioxidant.
- Omega-3 fats downregulate prostaglandin pathways that drive pain.
- Fiber supports estrogen clearance, digestive balance, and microbial diversity.

Healing does not happen through extremes. It happens through consistency — meals that calm the nervous system, supply nutrients for repair, and eliminate destabilizing spikes and crashes.

MACRONUTRIENT HARMONY AS DAILY SELF-REGULATION

A balanced meal is not only fuel; it is a message to the body that it is safe. Safety allows inflammation to quiet, hormones to regulate, digestion to stabilize, and the nervous system to rest. Food becomes a tool for self-regulation, not control.

When women eat with balance rather than restriction, healing becomes sustainable, cravings lose intensity, and health becomes predictable rather than mysterious.

Macronutrient harmony isn't a diet — it's how the body organizes itself into balance.

CHAPTER 11

UNDERSTANDING FODMAPS: A GENTLE, SCIENCE-BASED GUIDE TO REDUCING BLOATING AND CALMING YOUR GUT

Bloating, heaviness after meals, lower-belly pressure, unpredictable digestion — these symptoms can feel discouraging, especially when you're trying to eat "healthy." Many women spend years searching for answers, wondering why foods like apples, avocado, lentils, garlic, or cauliflower cause discomfort.

Your symptoms are not random. They follow a pattern. And one of the most powerful tools for uncovering that pattern is understanding FODMAPs.

WHAT FODMAPS ACTUALLY ARE

FODMAPs are short-chain carbohydrates found in many everyday foods. They are not "bad" or unsafe — many are deeply nutritious. The issue arises only when a sensitive or inflamed gut struggles to digest them.

Instead of being fully absorbed in the small intestine, they travel into the large intestine undigested. There, they ferment rapidly and draw water into the gut. This fermentation–fluid shift can cause:

- bloating
- distension or a visibly swollen belly
- pressure or cramping
- unpredictable bowel movements
- gas or heaviness after meals

Research from Monash University — the creators of the FODMAP protocol — shows that reducing these carbohydrates significantly decreases bloating and abdominal pain (Gibson & Shepherd, 2010). MRI studies confirm that high-FODMAP meals visibly increase gas and water content in sensitive individuals (Major et al., 2017).

The food isn't the problem. The current condition of your gut is.

WHAT "FODMAP" REALLY MEANS

The University of Virginia Digestive Health Center offers one of the clearest definitions. The acronym describes the carbohydrate groups most likely to trigger symptoms in a sensitive gut:

- **F — Fermentable**
  These carbohydrates quickly ferment in the gut, causing gas.
- **O — Oligosaccharides**
  Found in wheat, onions, garlic, beans, and legumes.
- **D — Disaccharides**
  Primarily lactose found in dairy.
- **M — Monosaccharides**
  Especially fructose in certain fruits and processed foods.
- **A — And**

- **P — Polyols**
  Sugar alcohols used in "sugar-free" products and naturally present in some fruits and vegetables.

When not properly absorbed, these carbohydrates move into the colon where they ferment rapidly. This fermentation is normal — but in a sensitive gut, it can create overwhelming pressure, bloating, gas, and discomfort.

This isn't about memorizing science. It's about recognizing that symptoms have logic — your gut is reacting to how these carbohydrates behave, not because something is "wrong" with you.

A HIDDEN REALITY: IBS IS OFTEN UNDIAGNOSED

Many assume FODMAP sensitivity only applies to people diagnosed with IBS. In reality, IBS is widely underdiagnosed — especially in women. Up to 70% of people with IBS-like symptoms never receive an official diagnosis (Lovell & Ford, 2012).

Symptoms are frequently dismissed, fluctuate with hormones, or appear "normal" on tests, leaving many women without answers.

Even more importantly, UVA's 2023 guidelines note that people without IBS can still experience strong reactions to FODMAPs. Sensitivity is common in women with:

- endometriosis
- PCOS
- chronic inflammation
- autoimmune tendencies
- hormonal fluctuations
- high stress or anxiety

- post-antibiotic microbiome disruption
- a "normal" colonoscopy

MRI studies confirm that even individuals without IBS can experience distension, gas, and fermentation after high-FODMAP meals (Marciani et al., 2010).

Your symptoms are real. Your body is communicating — and now you understand the language.

WHY WOMEN ARE MORE SENSITIVE TO FODMAPS

Women's digestive systems change throughout the menstrual cycle. Research in *Neurogastroenterology & Motility* shows that:

- pelvic nerves are more sensitive at certain times of the cycle
- estrogen and progesterone influence gut motility
- inflammation increases digestive reactivity
- stress heightens visceral sensitivity (Heitkemper & Chang, 2009)

This is why bloating often worsens:

- before menstruation
- during ovulation
- during periods of high stress

It is not in your head. It is rooted in biology.

THE THREE-PHASE FODMAP METHOD

Clinically validated and effective for reducing bloating, distension, and discomfort.

Phase 1 – Calming (2–6 weeks)

A temporary reduction of high-FODMAP foods to allow the gut to settle. Clinical studies show that 70–75% of people experience symptom improvement (Staudacher et al., 2011). Many women feel lighter within days.

Phase 2 – Reintroduction

This phase reveals your unique patterns. You reintroduce foods one by one to see:

- which categories you tolerate
- which cause mild symptoms
- which create strong reactions
- how portion size affects your body

You may tolerate apples but not garlic.
Avocado may feel fine in small amounts but not large portions.
You might handle chickpeas — but only half a cup.

This is personalized medicine you can do yourself.

Phase 3 – Personalized Eating (Your Long-Term Rhythm)

You are no longer avoiding foods — you understand your body.

You learn:

- how much you can tolerate
- when to eat more gently (PMS, stress, travel)

- which foods nourish you
- which feel heavy or overwhelming

Monash and UVA emphasize: flexibility, not avoidance, is the goal.

HIGH-FODMAP FOODS THAT COMMONLY TRIGGER SYMPTOMS

Common triggers include:

- **Fruits:** apples, pears, watermelon, cherries, mango
- **Vegetables:** onions, garlic, mushrooms, cauliflower, asparagus
- **Legumes and beans**
- **Grains:** wheat, barley, rye
- **Sweeteners and dairy:** honey and lactose-containing dairy
- **Sugar alcohols:** xylitol, sorbitol, mannitol, maltitol

However, tolerance varies dramatically. Reintroduction reveals how your gut responds — not general rules.

FODMAP-FRIENDLY FOODS THAT CALM THE GUT

Gentle, nourishing options include:

- berries, kiwi, pineapple, grapes, citrus
- zucchini, spinach, pumpkin, carrots, peppers
- rice, oats, quinoa, buckwheat
- almond milk, lactose-free milk, firm cheeses (if tolerated)
- maple syrup, pure stevia

These foods soothe digestion without starving the microbiome or triggering fermentation overload.

COMMON MISTAKES WOMEN MAKE (AND HOW TO AVOID THEM)

- **Staying low-FODMAP too long** → reduces microbiome diversity, worsens symptoms over time.
- **Reintroducing too quickly** → the gut needs clarity, not chaos.
- **Stacking multiple moderate-FODMAP foods** → even tolerated foods can overwhelm the gut when combined.
- **Ignoring hormones or stress** → cortisol and PMS amplify FODMAP reactions.
- **Skipping meals or eating too fast** → weakens digestion and increases sensitivity.

Healing requires gentleness, not perfection.

TRACKING SYMPTOMS WITHOUT ANXIETY

Your journal should feel supportive, not restrictive. Track only:

- what you ate
- how you felt 1–3 hours later
- stress level
- cycle phase

Patterns emerge naturally and without pressure.

WHAT HAPPENS WHEN THE GUT HEALS

As inflammation decreases and the microbiome strengthens:

- fermentation becomes milder
- bloating decreases
- food tolerance widens
- bowel movements become more regular

- nerve sensitivity calms

Many women gradually regain tolerance for:

- garlic and onions
- apples and avocado
- legumes
- cauliflower and mushrooms

Healing is not linear, but it is absolutely possible.

YOUR BODY IS NOT DIFFICULT – IT'S COMMUNICATING

When you understand FODMAPs, you stop blaming yourself for digestive symptoms. You begin to see the logic behind them.

As UVA's digestive team notes: relief comes not from restriction, but from understanding.

Your gut is not your enemy. It is your teacher, your guide, and your messenger. And now, you know how to listen.

CHAPTER 12

INTERMITTENT FASTING FOR WOMEN: A GENTLE, SCIENCE-BASED FRAMEWORK

Intermittent fasting can be a powerful tool for lowering inflammation, improving metabolic health, supporting digestion, and stabilizing energy. But women do not respond to fasting the same way men do. Female hormones, stress pathways, and the nervous system are more sensitive to calorie timing and prolonged fasting windows.

For women, the goal is not to push the body. The goal is to support biological rhythm.

Fasting works best when it **reduces metabolic burden** without increasing stress. This chapter explains how to use fasting in a way that is effective, sustainable, and hormonally safe.

WHY FASTING HELPS INFLAMMATION

When digestion rests, several beneficial processes become more active:

- **Improved insulin sensitivity**, leading to more stable blood sugar
- **Lower inflammatory signaling**, including reductions in IL-6 and TNF-α
- **Enhanced cellular cleanup (autophagy)**
- **Improved mitochondrial efficiency**, supporting energy and metabolism
- **Better gut motility**, allowing the digestive tract to reset

These changes support healing in conditions like endometriosis, PCOS, IBS, autoimmune tendencies, and chronic fatigue—but only when fasting is done in a way that respects hormonal needs.

WHY WOMEN NEED A DIFFERENT APPROACH

Women are more sensitive to deep caloric deficits and long fasting windows. Excessive fasting can:

- disrupt ovulation
- increase cortisol
- destabilize blood sugar
- worsen PMS
- trigger anxiety or sleep issues
- increase inflammation through stress pathways

A female-aligned fasting protocol focuses on **short, consistent fasts** and **biological feedback**, not extremes.

THE FOUNDATION: DAILY 12–13 HOUR FAST (MOST EFFECTIVE & SAFEST)

Most women benefit from a simple overnight fast:

12–13 hours without food
Example: finish eating at 7 pm → breakfast at 7–8 am.

This window:

- supports gut repair
- lowers nighttime inflammation
- stabilizes circadian rhythm
- improves digestion
- does not elevate cortisol

This is the baseline for everyone unless medically contraindicated.

THE OPTIONAL EXTENSION: 14–16 HOUR FAST (ONLY ON SPECIFIC DAYS)

Some women feel well extending their overnight fast a few times per week:

14–16 hours
Example: finish eating at 7 pm → first meal at 9–11 am.

Choose these days when:

- sleep was good
- stress is low
- energy is steady
- you are not in PMS or menstruation
- you feel strong, not depleted

Signs you should *shorten* the fast:

- anxiety
- irritability
- dizziness
- poor sleep
- extreme hunger
- PMS worsening

Fasting must adapt to biology—not the other way around.

FASTING ACROSS THE MENSTRUAL CYCLE

Your hormonal needs change weekly. Fasting should change with them.

Menstrual Phase

Avoid long fasting windows. Prioritize warm, frequent meals.
A gentle 12-hour fast is ideal.

Follicular Phase

Estrogen rises → fasting tolerance is highest.
Optional 14–16 hour fasts can be introduced here.

Ovulatory Phase

Estrogen peaks. Stress sensitivity may increase.
Light fasting (12–14 hours) is usually best.

Luteal Phase

Progesterone rises → metabolism increases.
Women genuinely need more calories and carbohydrates.
Limit fasting to 12–13 hours.

What to Consume During a Fast

Water, herbal tea, mineral-rich infusions, and diluted electrolytes are appropriate.
Avoid coffee on an empty stomach if you have anxiety, histamine issues, reflux, or blood sugar instability — caffeine spikes cortisol and can worsen symptoms.

BREAKING THE FAST

A protein-rich, warm meal regulates blood sugar and prevents cortisol spikes. Examples:

- chia pudding with berries and pumpkin seeds
- tofu scramble with spinach
- quinoa with tahini and fruit
- a smoothie with protein, berries, chia, and almond butter

Avoid breaking a fast with:

- fruit alone
- pastries
- coffee alone
- high-sugar foods

These destabilize blood sugar, increasing inflammation.

WHO SHOULD AVOID EXTENDED FASTING (BEYOND 12 HOURS)

- pregnancy or postpartum
- active eating disorders
- adrenal dysfunction
- hypothyroidism (untreated)

- severe PMS or PMDD
- underweight or chronically low appetite
- high stress, poor sleep, or intense training
- during illness or recovery

In these cases, gentle 12-hour overnight fasting is enough.

OPTIONAL TOOL: OCCASIONAL 24-HOUR FAST

A 24-hour fast is **not required** and **not appropriate for everyone**. But when done infrequently and safely, it can support:

- improved insulin sensitivity
- deeper autophagy
- digestive reset
- reduced inflammation
- metabolic clarity

How Often?

Once every 2–4 weeks, *only if you feel well.*

How to Structure It

The safest female-aligned version:

- Eat dinner at 6–7 pm
- Fast overnight + next day
- Hydrate with warm water, herbal tea, electrolytes
- End the fast with a warm, protein-rich meal the following evening

Avoid during:

- PMS
- menstruation
- high stress
- intense exercise periods
- poor sleep
- any sign of hormonal instability

A 24-hour fast should feel challenging but manageable — never extreme.

If you feel shaky, irritable, cold, anxious, or dizzy → end the fast. Your nervous system always outranks the protocol.

PLANT-BASED CONSIDERATIONS

Women following a plant-focused or fully plant-based diet often thrive on fasting when meals include:

- adequate protein (tofu, lentils, tempeh, pea protein, quinoa)
- enough healthy fats (chia, flax, hemp, walnuts, tahini)
- stable carbohydrates (sweet potato, oats, rice, legumes)

Fasting should **not** be used to compensate for undereating.
A nutritionally complete diet is essential before extending fasts.

HOW TO KNOW FASTING IS WORKING

Benefits appear gradually:

- clearer thinking
- more stable blood sugar
- reduced bloating

- improved digestion
- calmer PMS
- more predictable energy
- lower inflammatory flare-ups

You should feel **supported**, not depleted.

HOW TO KNOW YOU NEED TO ADJUST

If fasting worsens:

- insomnia
- anxiety
- cravings
- irritability
- headaches
- cycle dysregulation
- fatigue

→ shorten the fasting window
→ increase food quality
→ add more protein and carbohydrates
→ evaluate stress and sleep

Fasting is a tool — not an obligation.

CLOSING SUMMARY

Intermittent fasting can be an effective part of an anti-inflammatory lifestyle when practiced with awareness, flexibility, and respect for hormonal needs. Most women benefit most from consistent 12–13 hour overnight fasts, with optional 14–16 hour fasts during low-stress phases of the cycle. Occasional 24-hour fasts may be helpful for some, but they are never required and must be approached thoughtfully.

Fasting should never strain the body or elevate stress. When used appropriately, it supports metabolic balance, calmer digestion, improved hormonal stability, and reduced inflammation. The purpose is not restriction — it is regulation. Fasting works best when it enhances safety, stability, and nourishment, allowing the body to heal without pressure or extremes.

CHAPTER 13

HEALING FOODS FOR CHRONIC INFLAMMATION

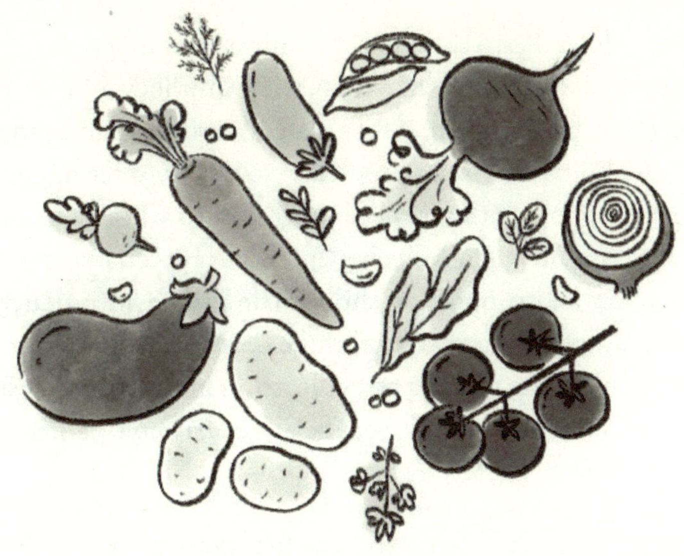

When the body is inflamed, it does not need restriction or control — it needs nourishment that calms the immune system, stabilizes hormones, supports digestion, clears toxins, and signals safety. Healing foods do not force change; they create the conditions in which change happens naturally.

Research shows that nutrient-dense, fiber-rich, polyphenol-rich, and omega-3–rich plant foods reduce inflammatory markers and support hormone balance, especially in women with endometriosis, PCOS, thyroid disorders, IBS, and metabolic inflammation (De Filippis et al., 2018; Schwingshackl et al., 2021). Healing happens most consistently through rhythm — not intensity or perfection.

Below are foods that communicate safety, reduce inflammation, and support deep biological repair.

Japanese Purple Sweet Potatoes

Their deep violet flesh comes from anthocyanins — the same potent antioxidants found in blueberries. Anthocyanins reduce oxidative stress, help regulate inflammatory pathways, and support metabolic stability. These potatoes digest slowly, offering steady blood sugar support without the sharp rise seen with white potatoes. Their resistant starch feeds beneficial gut bacteria, improving bowel function and supporting short-chain fatty acid production — a crucial process for gut and immune health. Resistant starch is a type of carbohydrate that bypasses digestion in the small intestine and becomes nourishment for beneficial gut bacteria, rather than raising blood sugar.

The Okinawan population, known for exceptional longevity, consumed these potatoes as a staple, associating them with metabolic resilience and low rates of inflammatory disease. Roasted or steamed with extra-virgin olive oil, they are both comforting and deeply nourishing, supporting hormonal balance and skin health through vitamin C–driven collagen support.

Chia and Flax Seeds

Chia and flax contain anti-inflammatory omega-3 fatty acids, lignans (which support estrogen metabolism), and soothing soluble fiber. Their gel-like texture when soaked coats and calms the intestinal lining, making them helpful for IBS, gastritis, and post-antibiotic recovery. Omega-3s also act on prostaglandins, which influence menstrual pain. For best absorption, flaxseed should be freshly ground; chia should be soaked before eating.

Lentils and Legumes

Lentils are an accessible source of fiber and plant protein, supporting blood sugar stability, digestive motility, hormone metabolism, and long-term satiety. Their prebiotic fiber feeds gut bacteria that produce anti-inflammatory short-chain fatty acids. For women with IBS or histamine sensitivity, lentils may be better tolerated than chickpeas, especially when soaked, rinsed well, and cooked thoroughly. Small portions with herbs or olive oil offer steady nourishment without heaviness.

Quinoa

Quinoa is a complete protein containing all essential amino acids, making it especially supportive during inflammation and menstrual recovery. Unlike many grains, quinoa has a gentle effect on blood sugar and is rich in magnesium — a mineral that relaxes muscles, calms the nervous system, supports sleep quality, and aids progesterone balance. When rinsed and cooked well, quinoa is soothing for the gut and appropriate for flare days and fatigue.

Medicinal Mushrooms

Shiitake, maitake, oyster, and lion's mane mushrooms contain beta-glucans — natural compounds that regulate immune responses without overstimulation. They support microbiome diversity and reduce inflammatory markers (Jayachandran et al., 2017). Mushrooms are grounding foods: mineral-rich, low-glycemic, and supportive for women with autoimmunity or pelvic inflammation. Lightly sautéed with olive oil or simmered into broth, they offer deep nourishment without intensity.

Aloe Vera

Aloe vera gel soothes the gastric and intestinal lining, making it beneficial for IBS, reflux, and inflammatory gut conditions. Its polysaccharides support mucosal healing and hydration from within. Aloe can also soften histamine irritation when the gut lining is compromised. Only inner gel should be consumed; the outer rind contains stimulating compounds that may irritate sensitive digestion.

Extra-Virgin Olive Oil (EVOO)

True EVOO is cold-pressed, unrefined, and rich in polyphenols — compounds that protect blood vessels, reduce oxidative stress, and support hormonal metabolism. Unlike refined oils, EVOO retains antioxidant potency, which influences pain pathways similarly to mild NSAIDs due to oleocanthal content (Parkinson & Cicerale, 2016). The slight burning sensation in the throat when tasting high-quality EVOO is a sign of these active compounds. Used daily — drizzled on warm vegetables, lentils, quinoa, or added at the end of cooking — EVOO supports menstrual comfort, cardiovascular health, metabolic resilience, and glowing skin.

ANTI-INFLAMMATORY FATS: NUTS & SEEDS

Nuts and seeds deliver healthy fats, protein, antioxidants, and minerals that support hormones, gut health, the nervous system, and skin integrity. Walnuts provide plant-based omega-3s that reduce inflammatory signaling. Almonds and sunflower seeds supply vitamin E that protects cell membranes and supports skin repair. Pumpkin seeds offer zinc and magnesium, crucial for progesterone production, stress regulation, and menstrual balance. Brazil nuts provide selenium for thyroid function, which influences metabolism, cycle regularity, and emotional stability. Pistachios contain lutein and polyphenols that support vascular health and reduce inflammatory oxidative stress. Hemp seeds supply complete protein and are well tolerated even by those with digestive sensitivity.

These foods are potent, so small daily servings — a handful of nuts or two to three tablespoons of seeds — deliver benefits without overwhelming digestion.

MINERAL-RICH HORMONE STABILIZERS

Minerals are deeply involved in hormone synthesis, detoxification, thyroid function, mood, and blood sugar stabilization. Seaweed delivers iodine and trace minerals essential for thyroid hormones, which regulate menstrual health, mood, temperature regulation, and metabolic rate. Pumpkin seeds, cashews, and lentils provide zinc and magnesium needed for progesterone balance, stable blood sugar, and calmer nervous-system signaling. Brazil nuts offer selenium that protects the thyroid from oxidative stress and supports immune resilience.

These foods act like nutritional messengers, supporting hormonal communication and metabolic rhythm without the need for supplementation when eaten consistently.

GENTLE FRUIT ALLIES FOR INFLAMED DIGESTION

Fruit can be healing when digestion is sensitive — if the right fruits are chosen. Dragon fruit is soothing, mineral-rich, and rich in soft prebiotics that feed beneficial bacteria without provoking fermentation. Pomegranate offers polyphenols that reduce oxidative stress, support blood vessels, and help the liver metabolize estrogen more efficiently, easing PMS heaviness and pelvic discomfort. Persimmon is naturally low in acidity, gentle on the gut, and provides slow-release carbohydrates that steady energy without irritation. Blueberries deliver anthocyanins that protect against oxidative stress and inflammation while remaining friendly to IBS when eaten fresh rather than dried.

These fruits provide nourishment without overstimulation — ideal for flare days or when digestion feels unpredictable.

Sidebar: For IBS and Histamine Sensitivity

Start small and pair with protection.
Begin with modest portions and combine them with soothing supports such as aloe gel, chamomile tea, chia pudding, or extra-virgin olive oil.

Fermented foods and leftovers need timing.
Enjoy fermented foods only in small amounts and ideally on days when you are not eating other high-histamine foods. Freshly cooked meals are usually easier to tolerate than leftovers.

Seeds require preparation.
Flax should be freshly ground; chia should be soaked. Unprepared seeds can irritate the gut lining when digestion is compromised.

DAO can offer temporary support.
During flare-ups, a DAO supplement before meals can help break down dietary histamine. This is not a long-term solution — it simply reduces symptoms while the gut heals.

Add, don't restrict.
Focus on adding soothing foods first. As the gut heals, tolerance naturally expands without elimination diets.

Creating a Healing Rhythm

The most powerful part of these foods is not their individuality, but their consistency. When eaten regularly, they support liver detoxification, regulate estrogen and progesterone balance, nourish gut bacteria, stabilize blood sugar, reduce oxidative stress, and calm immune overactivity. Healing foods work the way the body does: slowly, rhythmically, intentionally. They become nourishment, not restriction; clarity, not confusion; support, not pressure.

In this rhythm, food stops being the enemy and becomes something more intimate — a tool for biological peace.

CHAPTER 14

ADAPTOGENS: NATURE'S ALLIES FOR STRESS, ENERGY & HORMONAL BALANCE

Modern life keeps the body in a state of urgency. We wake to notifications, rush through tasks, push ourselves to perform, and fall asleep with thoughts still spinning. The nervous system, designed for rhythm and recovery, rarely receives the message that it is safe. When stress becomes constant, cortisol rises, digestion weakens, hormones destabilize, inflammation increases, and energy becomes unpredictable.

Adaptogens are plants and mushrooms that help the body adapt to stress rather than collapse under it. They influence the hypothalamic–pituitary–adrenal (HPA) axis — the communication loop between the brain and adrenal glands that regulates cortisol, mood, focus, immune activity, and metabolic resilience. When this system becomes strained, the body reacts emotionally, hormonally, and physically. Adaptogens do not stimulate or sedate; they help restore equilibrium.

Their medicine is slow, cumulative, and intelligent. They are not quick fixes. They work gently over time, as daily allies that rebuild depleted energy, support hormonal balance, and strengthen nervous-system stability.

SAFETY FIRST: READ BEFORE USING ADAPTOGENS

Adaptogens can influence hormones, thyroid function, neurotransmitters, liver detoxification, blood pressure, and immune activity. Because of this, they may interact with medications or existing medical conditions.

Seek medical guidance before using adaptogens if you are:

- Taking antidepressants (SSRIs/SNRIs), mood stabilizers, or antipsychotics
- Using hormonal treatments or birth control
- Taking thyroid medication
- Using blood thinners, blood pressure medication, steroids, or diabetic medication (including metformin)
- Pregnant, breastfeeding, or trying to conceive
- Living with hypertension, heart conditions, kidney disease, or autoimmune disorders under treatment

Avoid without supervision:

- **Licorice root**
- **Shilajit**
- **Ceremonial herbs (e.g., blue lotus)** when on psychiatric medication or during trauma recovery

Adaptogens are powerful. Respect them. They should be used as part of a healing plan, not randomly added to a routine.

CALMING ADAPTOGENS: FOR ANXIETY, REST, AND EMOTIONAL OVERWHELM

These herbs help quiet overstimulation and reduce cortisol, allowing the nervous system to feel safe again. They are especially supportive when anxiety is paired with fatigue, irritability, insomnia, or "wired but tired" energy.

Ashwagandha

A deeply grounding Ayurvedic root that regulates cortisol, supports sleep quality, calms anxiety, and eases PMS mood swings. It can also stabilize thyroid function when stress is the root of imbalance. For many women, it becomes the foundation of nervous-system repair.

Reishi Mushroom

Known as the "mushroom of calm," reishi contains triterpenes that relax the nervous system and beta-glucans that reduce inflammation. It supports immune health without stimulation and improves sleep depth. Reishi can also ease histamine-related inflammation when the gut begins to heal.

Tulsi (Holy Basil)

Tulsi reduces cortisol and stabilizes blood sugar fluctuations driven by stress. As a tea, it works gently and consistently, helping calm tension in the chest, jaw, and digestive system. Especially helpful for stress-induced bloating, emotional overwhelm, and anxious digestion.

Supportive Options

Maca and *Schisandra* may be calming or energizing depending on the individual. They are best introduced later, after core stabilization with the adaptogens above.

ENERGIZING ADAPTOGENS: FOR FATIGUE, BRAIN FOG, AND MOTIVATION

These herbs support stamina without stimulation. They enhance oxygen use, mitochondrial energy, and cognitive focus — ideal when fatigue is mental, not emotional.

Rhodiola Rosea
A powerful Arctic root that sharpens concentration, improves mood, and increases stress resilience. Best for burnout-related fatigue and mental exhaustion. Not recommended when anxiety is severe unless guided by a practitioner.

Panax Ginseng (Asian Ginseng)
Supports mitochondrial energy, circulation, and stamina. Its effect builds slowly, providing steady strength rather than a "boost." Not ideal for women with uncontrolled high blood pressure.

Cordyceps Mushroom
Enhances oxygen absorption and ATP production — the body's cellular energy. Traditionally used after illness, chronic fatigue, or physical depletion. Cordyceps is especially helpful when routine tasks feel draining (e.g., climbing stairs, standing too long).

Supportive Options
Eleuthero (Siberian Ginseng) is gentler and good for gradual recovery. **Shilajit requires medical supervision due to risk of heavy metal contamination.**

ADAPTOGENS FOR HORMONES & IMMUNE BALANCE

These herbs support liver detoxification, estrogen metabolism, collagen repair, immune regulation, and menstrual rhythm. Ideal for estrogen dominance, PMS, skin inflammation, and immune-related fatigue.

Schisandra Berry
A liver-supporting adaptogen that helps metabolize estrogen, reduce PMS heaviness, and brighten skin. Enhances focus and stamina without stimulation. Supports collagen preservation during stress.

Astragalus Root
Strengthens connective tissue, supports immune balance, and gently detoxifies the body. Particularly helpful for women who have depleted immunity due to chronic stress.

Amla (Indian Gooseberry)
Rich in vitamin C and antioxidants that support hormonal balance, collagen production, skin clarity, and anti-inflammatory protection. Ideal for dull skin, brittle hair, fatigue around menstruation, and slow cycle recovery.

Use With Caution

Licorice Root calms the adrenal response and repairs the gut lining, but can alter blood pressure, potassium levels, and hormone metabolism. Use only with professional supervision.

HOW TO USE ADAPTOGENS WISELY

Healing happens in rhythm, not intensity.

Guidelines:

- Introduce **one adaptogen at a time** for 3–4 weeks before adding another.
- Avoid continuous use; after 8–12 weeks, **pause for 2–4 weeks** or rotate.

- Small daily amounts are more effective than high doses.
- Pair with lifestyle: sleep, nourishing meals, stress regulation, gut healing.
- Choose high-quality sources with no fillers, artificial flavors, or contamination.

ALIGNING ADAPTOGENS WITH THE MENSTRUAL CYCLE

Supporting herbs based on cyclical needs helps stabilize hormones more naturally.

Follicular Phase (after menstruation)
Rhodiola or Tulsi for clarity, motivation, and stable energy.

Ovulation
Schisandra or Maca to support vitality, libido, and skin radiance.

Luteal Phase (before menstruation)
Ashwagandha or Reishi to ease irritability, PMS mood shifts, bloating, and inflammation.

Menstruation
Reishi, Tulsi, or (with supervision) Licorice root for rest, repair, and digestive ease.

This rhythm mirrors what the body is designed for — **changing needs, changing support.**

EMOTIONAL & CEREMONIAL HERBS (OPTIONAL)

These herbs influence emotional presence more than hormonal or metabolic repair. They are useful for mindfulness, creative processing, breathwork, and internal reflection.

Blue Lotus
Traditionally used to quiet the mind and deepen meditation. Avoid when using psychiatric medication.

Damiana
Supports relaxation, sensuality, and emotional confidence. May interact with antidepressants or hormonal medications.

Rose
Gentle and safe when used as tea or aromatherapy. Helps soften emotional tension and support emotional expression.

These plants offer emotional grounding — not clinical adaptogenic effects.

THE MEDICINE OF BALANCE

Adaptogens do not force the body into change. They teach it how to find equilibrium again. True resilience is not speed, intensity, or pushing harder. It is rhythm, nourishment, and a nervous system that no longer believes it must survive every minute.

When life becomes too loud, adaptogens remind the body that strength comes from safety.

Resilience is not doing more.
It is doing what supports peace.

PART IV

LIFESTYLE & EMOTIONAL HEALING: CREATING SAFETY IN THE BODY

CHAPTER 15

CALMING THE FIRE: WHEN SAFETY BECOMES MEDICINE

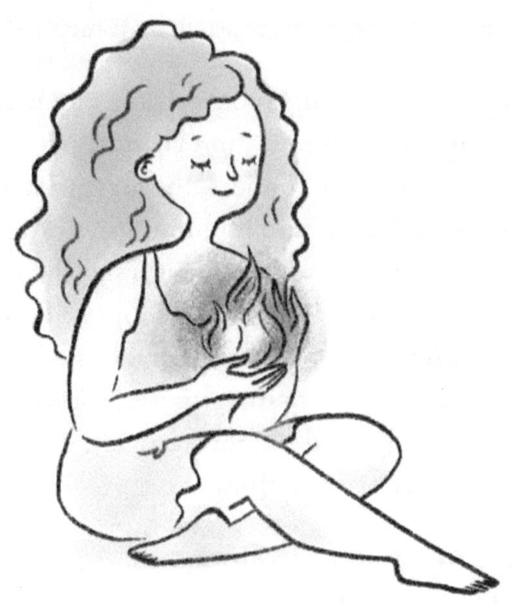

Nutrition is only one part of recovery from chronic inflammation. Even the most carefully designed anti-inflammatory diet cannot fully repair a body that remains in a state of survival.

The nervous system must experience safety for hormones to regulate, digestion to normalize, and pain signals to quiet. Healing is not only about what is eaten, but also about how the body rests, breathes, and perceives its environment.

When the brain interprets stress—whether physical, emotional, or cognitive—it signals the release of cortisol and adrenaline. Short bursts of these hormones help the body respond to immediate challenges. When stress becomes continuous, the same responses that once protected the body begin to inflame it. The nervous system remains alert, immune cells stay activated, digestion slows, and inflammatory pathways remain elevated. In this state, healing becomes biologically difficult, not because the body is weak, but because it believes it must protect rather than repair.

A key pathway involved in this process is the **vagus nerve.** Often described as the main communication channel between the brain and the body, the vagus nerve connects the nervous system with the heart, lungs, digestive organs, and immune system. When the body remains in a prolonged stress response, vagal signaling becomes less effective, and processes such as digestion, immune balance, and tissue repair can be disrupted. When the nervous system experiences safety and regulation, vagal activity improves, allowing the body to shift out of survival mode and support recovery, digestion, and the resolution of inflammatory responses.

The body has two major nervous system states that strongly influence inflammation, digestion, hormone balance, and healing: the sympathetic state of protection and the parasympathetic state of restoration.

The parasympathetic nervous system is often described as the body's "rest, digest, and repair" mode. This is where heart rate slows, digestion improves, stress hormones begin to regulate, and the body can redirect energy toward tissue repair, immune balance, and hormonal stability. A central part of this process is the vagus nerve, which plays a key role in helping the body return to this restorative state.

The goal is not to eliminate stress completely, but to regularly guide the body back into safety. Even small, consistent signals of calm can begin to shift the nervous system toward healing.

Modern life is often fast-paced, demanding, and overstimulating. For many people, it may feel like a luxury to have time for a slow morning or to engage in mindful practices consistently. This is a common and understandable reality.

There are also many different approaches to supporting the nervous system, and each person may respond differently. What feels calming and effective for one person may not feel the same for another.

For this reason, it can be helpful to explore a few different practices and notice how your body responds. Even small, brief moments of regulation can be meaningful. The practices can be combined in ways that feel natural—for example, journaling in nature, listening to calming sounds during meditation, or pairing gentle movement with breathwork.

For some individuals, particularly women navigating chronic symptoms, there can be a tendency to feel discouraged or self-critical when routines are not followed perfectly. This pressure can unintentionally increase stress rather than support healing.

It is important to approach these tools with flexibility and self-awareness. Missing a day or not following a routine consistently is not a failure, and it does not undo progress.

In many cases, the most beneficial shift is not adding more practices, but changing the way we relate to ourselves. Speaking internally with patience, understanding, and compassion—similar to how we would speak to someone we love—can have a profound effect on the nervous system.

Gentleness, consistency, and self-acceptance often support healing more effectively than pressure or perfection.

GENTLE PRACTICES THAT SUPPORT NERVOUS SYSTEM REGULATION

Slow, consistent practices send clear biological signals of safety. These practices influence inflammation not through belief alone, but through measurable effects on cortisol, vagal tone, immune signaling, and hormonal regulation.

Deep Breathing

Slow nasal breathing activates the vagus nerve, which lowers heart rate and reduces cortisol. Techniques such as the 4–7–8 breath (inhale for four, hold for seven, exhale for eight) can help calm the body's internal alarm system.

Start with 3–5 rounds once or twice daily, especially in the morning, before meals, or before sleep. Even a few minutes of slow breathing can begin shifting the body toward parasympathetic regulation.

Meditation and Stillness

Even brief periods of guided relaxation or quiet observation have been shown to reduce anxiety, support hormonal balance, and decrease inflammatory activity.

Meditation does not need to be long or complex. Starting with 5 minutes daily is enough to begin supporting nervous system regulation. Many people find it easiest to practice in the morning or before sleep using guided tools such as Calm, Headspace, or Insight Timer. With consistency, improvements in stress response and sleep are often noticed within 1–2 weeks.

In the beginning, it is very common to feel frustrated when the mind does not stay focused for the full 5–10 minutes. This is a normal part of the process. Meditation is not about eliminating thoughts—it is about learning how to gently return attention.

A 10-minute session may offer only a few seconds—or even a single minute—of true stillness in the beginning, and even that brief moment can be beneficial for the nervous system.

A helpful approach is to release the idea that meditation must be perfect. The real practice is the return.

One simple technique is to focus on a single image, such as a cloud floating in the sky. When thoughts arise, imagine them as passing clouds and gently move them aside with a quiet inner response: not now. The goal is not force, but gentle redirection—with patience, softness, and lightness.

Sound and Nervous System Regulation

Sound therapy is an ancient practice that uses vibration and frequency to support relaxation, balance, and overall well-being. Across cultures, sound has long been used to influence emotional and physiological states.

During a sound bath, a practitioner may use instruments such as gongs, singing bowls, or chimes while participants rest comfortably.

The repetitive tones and vibrations may help calm the mind, relax the body, and support a shift toward parasympathetic activity.

Some individuals report reduced stress, improved sleep, and an increased sense of calm with regular sound-based practices. While responses can vary, this may be a supportive tool for nervous system regulation.

Attending a guided sound session once per week for several weeks or months may allow the body to gradually respond and adapt. As stress levels improve, maintenance sessions once or twice per month may help sustain the benefits.

At home, listening to calming music, nature sounds, or sound-based meditations for 5–15 minutes, particularly in the evening, may also support relaxation and sleep.

Creative Expression and Nervous System Regulation

Creative activities such as drawing, painting, writing, or simple crafts can support nervous system balance. Engaging in creative expression shifts attention away from stress and into a focused, present-moment state.

For many individuals, the creative process becomes a form of meditation. It does not require artistic skill or perfection—the benefit comes from the act of creating.

Even 10–20 minutes of creative activity may help calm the mind, improve mood, and support emotional processing.

Body-Based Practices for Nervous System Regulation

The body and nervous system are closely connected. Certain physical positions and gentle movements can help signal safety and support parasympathetic activation.

One simple technique is the legs-up-the-wall position. Lie on your back with your legs resting vertically against a wall, allow your arms to rest comfortably, and remain in this position for 5–10 minutes while breathing slowly.

This may help reduce tension, support circulation, and encourage a shift into a more restorative state.

EFT Tapping (Emotional Freedom Technique)

EFT combines gentle tapping on acupressure points with focused attention on emotional or physical sensations. It may help reduce cortisol, regulate emotional stress, and influence how the brain processes pain and threat signals (Stapleton et al., 2022).

The following is an example of a tapping sequence. You may adapt the words and phrases to reflect your own emotions, physical sensations, or intentions. There is no single correct way to practice—what matters most is that the language feels supportive and authentic to you.

Example Tapping Ritual for Calm, Safety, and Healing

Find a quiet space and sit comfortably. Close your eyes and take three slow, deep breaths.

Set an intention:
I am here to calm my body, clear my mind, and invite healing, love, and ease.

Using your index and middle fingers, begin tapping gently at approximately one tap per second.

Tapping points: side of the hand, eyebrow, side of eye, under eye, under nose, chin, collarbone, under arm, top of head.

Setup statements:
Even though I sometimes feel pain, tension, and fear in my body, I deeply and completely accept myself.
Even though I have been through so much, I choose peace and healing.

Even though anxiety and uncertainty arise, I am learning to feel safe in my body again.

Tapping sequence (1–3 rounds):
Eyebrow: This pain, this inflammation, this tension in my body.
Side of eye: I have carried it for so long.
Under eye: It is safe now to release what no longer serves me.
Under nose: My body is learning peace.
Chin: I am healing.
Collarbone: Every cell in me is returning to balance.
Under arm: I am worthy of comfort, safety, and calm.
Top of head: I welcome lightness, balance, and healing.

Reframe round:
Eyebrow: My body is strong, wise, and resilient.
Side of eye: Healing flows through me with ease.
Under eye: I release resistance to feeling better.
Under nose: I am open to restoration and balance.
Chin: I welcome support in my healing.

Collarbone: Every breath brings me closer to vitality.
Under arm: Peace and safety surround me.
Top of head: I am supported, healing, and thriving.

Closing:
Place your hands over your heart and take one slow breath.
I am safe. My body is healing. I am supported.

Sit quietly for a moment and allow the body to settle.

Journaling and Gratitude Practice

Journaling can support emotional regulation and nervous system balance. Writing down three or more things you are grateful for in the morning and evening can help shift attention toward stability and safety.

I have found it helpful not only to express emotions through writing, but also to gently shift the narrative of difficult experiences. While writing about emotions can be beneficial, repeatedly focusing on the same negative experience without reframing it may reinforce stress responses.

On more difficult days, identifying even small moments of comfort can help regulate emotional responses and reduce perceived stress.

Technology Use and Nervous System Overload

Modern technology and constant digital stimulation can keep the nervous system in a state of alertness. Creating intentional breaks from screens may support focus, emotional balance, and overall nervous system regulation.

Simple practices can include limiting screen exposure before sleep, scheduling short periods without phone use, and reducing non-essential notifications.

The nervous system responds to repetition. When the body is exposed to consistent signals of calm, it can gradually shift away from a prolonged stress response and toward a more regulated state.

Healing does not require perfect conditions, but rather enough moments of safety to support this shift over time.

Safety is not only a subjective feeling—it is also a biological state that can be reinforced through daily habits and supportive practices.

When the body receives consistent signals of rest, nourishment, and regulation, processes such as digestion, hormonal balance, and tissue repair can function more effectively.

Sustainable healing is not driven by intensity or perfection, but by consistency and the gradual creation of conditions in which the body no longer remains in a constant state of defense.

CHAPTER 16

THE BODY REMEMBERS SAFETY: NATURE, RHYTHM & CONNECTION

Nutrition builds the foundation of healing, but safety completes it. Food can quiet inflammation, yet the nervous system determines whether the body repairs or stays in defense. True healing begins when biology stops bracing for danger.

Stress, pain, perfectionism, trauma, loneliness, comparison — these can keep the body in survival mode even when diet is perfect. Healing practices are not hobbies or "extras." They are biological interventions. They shift the body from defense into repair. They remind the brain and immune system that life does not have to be fought — it can be lived.

This chapter explores natural therapies that calm inflammation and restore harmony: grounding, forest immersion, sound healing, movement, journaling, rest, and human connection. None of these replace medical care or nutrition. They amplify it, supporting your biology instead of working against it.

Grounding: Reconnecting Body & Earth

Emerging research shows that direct skin contact with the Earth may lower inflammation, rebalance the nervous system, and support immune function (Menigoz et al., 2020). Grounding — such as standing barefoot on grass, soil, or sand — allows the body to exchange electrons with the Earth's natural electrical charge.

A review published in the *Journal of Inflammation Research* found that grounding can reduce pain, influence white-blood-cell behavior, and support wound healing through shifts in cytokine activity (Oschman, Chevalier & Brown, 2015).

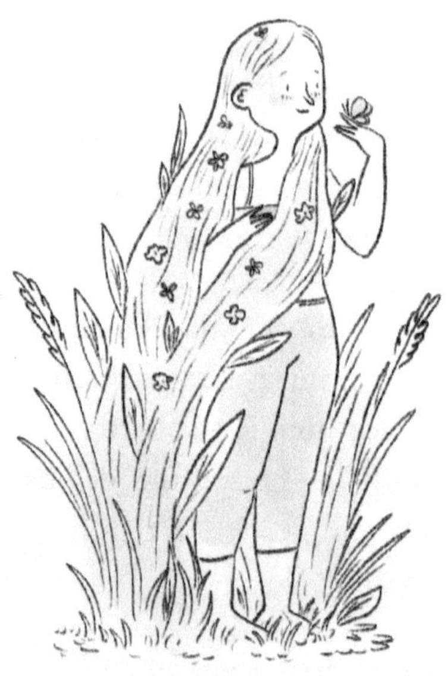

The mechanism is still being studied, but many people notice immediate effects: softer breath, calmer thoughts, deeper sleep, and less tension.

Grounding does not remove stress — it gives the body another source of support.

When paired with anti-inflammatory eating, grounding may enhance cellular repair, improve mood, and support energy.

Forest Bathing & Biophilia: Nature as Nervous System Therapy

If grounding is physical, forest immersion is sensory.
In Japan, doctors prescribe Shinrin-yoku — "forest bathing" — as therapy for stress and inflammation. Patients are encouraged to walk slowly, breathe deeply, and absorb nature through all senses: the sound of leaves, the smell of soil, the play of sunlight through branches.

Research shows that even 20 minutes in nature can lower cortisol, reduce inflammation, stabilize blood pressure, and support immune function. Western medicine now recognizes this. As Mayo Clinic's Dr. Brent Bauer explains:

"We are wired to be connected to nature… Research consistently shows drops in blood pressure and heart rate and overall wellbeing when we spend time in green environments." (Howland, 2024)

Nature does not demand productivity. It invites presence.
That alone is medicine.

Sound Therapy: Frequency as Cellular Communication

Sound changes brain waves. Vibrations from singing bowls, Tibetan bells, or even soft instrumental music help shift the brain into slower, restorative rhythms. This helps reduce cortisol, relax muscles, and release endorphins — natural pain and mood regulators.

A study found that a single sound meditation session significantly reduced anxiety, tension, fatigue, and even physical pain (Goldsby et al., 2016).

Soft sound is not entertainment. It is biological communication. It helps the nervous system remember how to rest.

In my own life, weekly sound baths helped reduce anxiety, soften inflammation, and stabilize mood — not overnight, but slowly, cumulatively. Sound works like nature does: quietly and deeply.

Movement as Medicine

Complete rest often worsens inflammation more than gentle movement. Light, calming activity increases lymphatic flow — the body's detox system — helping remove inflammatory waste (Li et al., 2023). Even slow stretching or walking releases myokines, signaling molecules that reduce inflammatory cytokines and support immune regulation (Pedersen & Saltin, 2015).

Some of the most healing forms of exercise are slow:

- Yoga Nidra (deep nervous system rest)
- Kundalini (breath and sound for release)
- Gentle Pilates
- Slow walking

Ask yourself:
"What is the smallest movement I can do today?"
Sometimes the smallest act creates the largest shift.

As a model, I once forced workouts no matter how I felt. It looked like discipline from the outside, but it was punishment. When movement comes from compassion instead of fear, the body responds with healing rather than resistance.

Journaling & Emotional Detox

Unexpressed emotions do not disappear. They become tension, inflammation, and pain stored in the body.
Writing freely — without rereading or editing — activates emotional-processing pathways in the brain and helps release latent stress. If writing feels difficult, drawing or coloring can offer the same release.

The goal isn't creativity — it's letting the body put something down.

Rest & Stillness

Stillness is different from sleep. It is a state of unproductive presence that serves a biological purpose. Sitting on a balcony without your phone, lying on the sofa without guilt, or quietly breathing in bed signals to your nervous system that nothing is required of you.

This increases vagal tone, lowers cortisol, and frees energy for repair. Rest is not a reward. It is treatment.

Connection, Safe Touch & Oxytocin

Oxytocin — the hormone of hugs, laughter, eye contact, pets, and emotional warmth — reduces cortisol, lowers inflammatory cytokines, and regulates pain.
Healing accelerates in safety and community. A supportive friend, a pet, a shared meal — these are not sentimental details. They are hormonal interventions.

Safety is shared.
The body heals more easily when it feels connected.

Creating a Personal Anti-Inflammatory Ritual

Healing is not about doing everything — it's about doing **a few things consistently**. Choose one or two practices that feel nourishing, not forced.

Example:

- **Morning:** 3 minutes of breath + gratitude journaling
- **Midday:** slow walk or gentle stretch
- **Evening:** herbal tea + soft sound or balcony stillness

Repetition teaches the nervous system a new language:
You are safe now. You can heal.

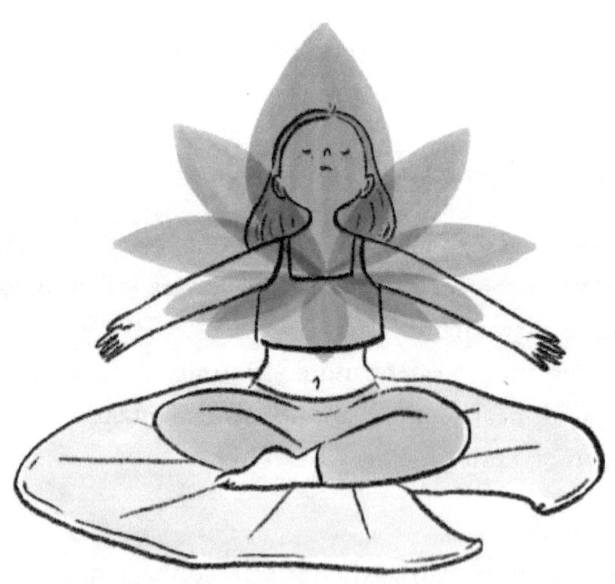

Closing Reflection

You cannot control every source of inflammation.
But you can control the environment inside your body.

Peace, rest, nature, and connection are not passive — they are active therapies.
When you nurture calm, inflammation loses its fuel.

Healing begins where it was once disrupted:
in breath, presence, softness, and the decision to let your body feel safe again.

CHAPTER 17

SLEEP IS WHERE THE BODY REPAIRS

Sleep is not passive. It is not "time off."
Sleep is the most active healing state the body ever enters.

During sleep, inflammation quiets, hormones recalibrate, immune cells repair tissue, and mitochondria restore energy production. For women living with chronic illness, hormonal imbalance, or persistent pain, sleep is not optional self-care — it is medicine.

Yet sleep is often the first thing we sacrifice. We stay up scrolling, worrying, or pushing productivity later into the night, believing we will recover tomorrow. But the body does not heal in fragments. It heals in rhythm.

Sleep, inflammation, and immune repair

Insufficient or fragmented sleep increases inflammatory activity and weakens immune regulation. Even short periods of poor sleep elevate inflammatory signaling, leaving tissues more reactive and less capable of repair. Neuroscientist Matthew Walker explains that sleep deprivation activates both stress and immune pathways simultaneously, creating a physiological environment in which inflammation is more easily triggered and more difficult to resolve (*Why We Sleep*).

For women with chronic illness, this connection is especially significant. When sleep is disrupted, the immune system remains in a low-grade defensive state. Pain feels sharper. Digestion becomes more reactive. Hormonal symptoms intensify. Sleep is not simply recovery from the day — it is the primary window in which inflammatory processes are actively dialed down. Without it, healing slows no matter how carefully other aspects of health are managed.

Sleep is the signal that danger has passed.

Sleep and pain perception

Pain is not only physical — it is neurological. The brain interprets and amplifies pain signals based on stress, safety, and exhaustion. Poor sleep lowers pain thresholds, making sensations that were once manageable feel overwhelming.

For women with endometriosis, fibromyalgia, migraines, IBS, or chronic pelvic pain, disrupted sleep can increase central sensitization — a state in which the nervous system becomes hyper-responsive. This does not mean pain is imagined. It means the brain is exhausted and less able to regulate incoming signals.

Restful sleep restores this regulation. It allows the nervous system to soften its grip, reducing the intensity and frequency of pain responses over time.

Why women often need more sleep

Sleep needs are not identical across sexes. Women, on average, require **slightly more sleep than men**, and this difference becomes more pronounced in the presence of hormonal fluctuation, inflammation, or chronic stress.

Hormones such as estrogen and progesterone interact directly with sleep architecture. They influence circadian rhythm, body temperature regulation, pain perception, and nervous system sensitivity. Across the menstrual cycle — and in conditions such as endometriosis or PCOS — the body often requires additional restorative time to regulate these systems.

Women also tend to have higher immune responsiveness. While this is protective, it increases physiological demand — and sleep is the primary window in which that demand is met.

This is not weakness.
It is biology.

How much sleep is ideal

Most adults function best with **7–9 hours of sleep** per night. For many women — especially those living with chronic illness, inflammation, or hormonal imbalance — the ideal range often falls toward the **upper end**, around **8–9 hours**.

Needing more sleep does not mean something is wrong. It often means the body is actively repairing.

During flare-ups, periods of stress, or recovery, temporary increases in sleep need are normal and appropriate. The body uses sleep to stabilize blood sugar, reduce pain sensitivity, regulate hormones, and restore immune balance. Shortening this process slows healing.

Rather than aiming for a rigid number, it is more helpful to notice how you feel:

- Is pain more manageable?
- Is mood steadier?
- Is energy more predictable?

These are signs that sleep is supporting you.

When sleep feels impossible

Sleep problems do not have a single cause. For many women with chronic illness, insomnia is not about poor habits or lack of discipline — it is a response to an overstimulated nervous system or a body in pain.

Some nights, the mind will not slow down. Thoughts race, worries surface, memories replay. Even when the body is exhausted, the brain remains alert.

Other nights, the issue is physical. Pain, bloating, pelvic tension, joint discomfort, or nerve sensitivity can make lying still unbearable. In these moments, sleep is not resisted — it is blocked by the body itself.

Both experiences are real.
Both deserve care.

Sleep difficulties are not a failure of willpower. They are signals of imbalance asking to be met with gentleness rather than force.

Supporting sleep when the mind won't quiet

When thoughts are the barrier, the goal is not to stop thinking, but to help the nervous system feel safe enough to soften.

Small sensory cues can help signal safety:

- dim lighting in the evening
- warm showers or baths
- consistent bedtime rituals

Magnesium taken in the evening can be especially supportive. Magnesium plays a role in nervous system regulation, muscle relaxation, and calming excitatory signals in the brain. Many women with chronic inflammation are deficient, and gentle supplementation at night often helps ease both mental tension and physical restlessness.

The intention is not sedation.
It is reassurance.

Supporting sleep when pain is the barrier

When pain prevents sleep, comfort becomes a medical need, not a luxury.

Lowering room temperature can significantly improve sleep quality. A slightly cooler environment supports melatonin production and aligns with the body's natural nighttime drop in core temperature.

Physical comfort matters:

- breathable bedding
- supportive pillows
- materials that reduce friction and irritation

Silk pillowcases and eye masks may seem small, but they can meaningfully reduce sensory input, facial tension, and skin irritation — especially for sensitive nervous systems.

Essential oils used subtly can also support relaxation. Scent communicates directly with emotional centers in the brain, bypassing analysis and signaling safety.

None of these tools are cures.
They are supports — ways of reducing friction so sleep has space to arrive.

Sound, familiarity, and calming the nervous system

Silence is not always soothing. For some nervous systems, quiet leaves space for discomfort or racing thoughts to intensify. Gentle, familiar sound can act as a bridge into sleep.

Listening to an audiobook you already know — one without suspense or emotional charge — reduces cognitive effort. Familiar narratives give the mind something predictable to rest against, allowing vigilance to soften. Walker notes that emotionally neutral, familiar sensory input helps the brain disengage from alertness and move toward rest.

Relaxing music can serve a similar role. Slow, repetitive rhythms and low stimulation support parasympathetic activation — the physiological state in which repair occurs.

Sound is not meant to overpower the body into sleep.
It is meant to accompany it.

Releasing pressure around sleep

One of the most overlooked contributors to insomnia is pressure. When sleep becomes another task to perform correctly, the nervous system remains alert.

If sleep does not come, rest still counts.

Lying quietly in darkness, breathing gently, allowing the body to be still — these moments reduce inflammatory load even without unconscious sleep. Healing occurs whenever the body feels safe, not only when sleep is perfect.

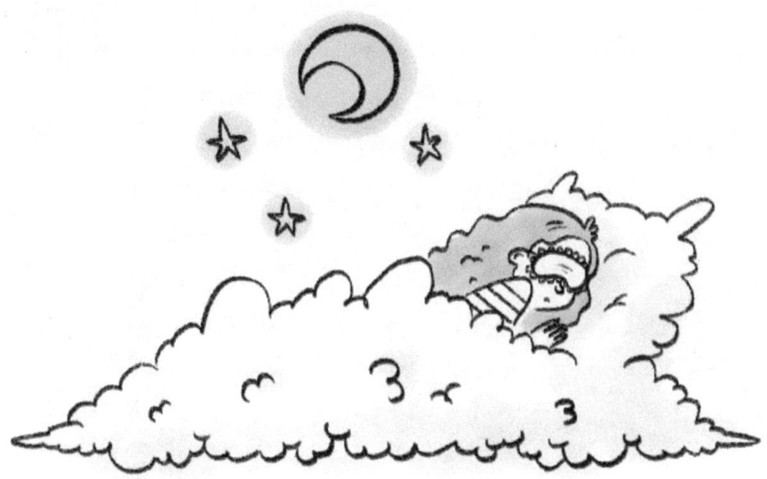

Some nights will be easier than others. That variability is part of healing, not evidence of failure.

You are not broken because sleep is hard.
Your body is asking for support — and support can be gentle.

CHAPTER 18

THE PATH FORWARD

Healing is not a moment — it is a rhythm.

After the urgency fades and the strict protocols soften, a new question appears:

How do I live like this long term?

The answer is integration.

Healing becomes sustainable not when it requires more effort but when it becomes a natural part of everyday life.

The goal is not perfection. It is awareness — noticing how your body responds, listening before it has to shout, returning to balance more easily each time you drift. Awareness becomes a compass. It guides your choices without obsession.

Healing as a Lifestyle, Not a Project

The practices that truly reshape health are simple, repeatable, and kind:

- morning light
- slow meals

- steady sleep
- daily breath
- movement that brings energy rather than drains it

These anchor the nervous system, stabilize blood sugar, improve hormone metabolism, and keep inflammation quiet. Complex protocols do not heal as deeply as consistent compassion.

Healing eventually stops being a task.
It becomes who you are.

Understanding Progress

Progress rarely looks linear. There will be light days and heavy days. Days when symptoms fade and days when they return. This rhythm is not failure — it is biology learning a new pattern.

Each time you recover from a flare, your nervous system "remembers" the path home.
When symptoms arise, ask gently:

"What might my body need today?"
Curiosity creates healing. Judgment inflames.

Creating Supportive Structure

Morning Grounding
Start the day with one intentional act before looking at your phone: a few breaths, a stretch, sunlight, or simply placing a hand on your heart. This small choice shapes cortisol rhythm for the entire day.

Nourishing Routine
Let food support you without dominating your life. Stock simple staples: greens, soups, smoothies, chia pudding, herbal teas. Healing meals can be effortless.

Digital Boundaries
Screens keep the stress response activated. Try screen-free meals, offline breaks, or a phone-free morning once a week.

Meaningful Movement
Move for energy, not performance. Match activity to your hormonal cycle and daily energy.

Connection and Community
Healing thrives in company. Share your experiences with people who understand chronic illness and holistic living. Support turns persistence into hope.

Nervous System Hygiene

Just as you clean your skin, the nervous system benefits from daily clearing:
deep breathing, a bath, journaling, soft music, stretching.
Preventive calm is an anti-inflammatory habit as real as nutrition or supplements.

Trusting Your Inner Compass

As the body heals, intuition sharpens. You'll begin to sense which foods nourish, which relationships elevate or deplete you, which environments feel safe. Listening to your body is not emotional — it is biological feedback. The nervous system stores memory through sensation.

Your body's wisdom is not dramatic; it is subtle and steady.

When Life Gets Busy Again

You will travel, work late, eat at restaurants, and experience stress. Healing does not ask you to avoid life — it equips you to live it better.

When life becomes chaotic, return to your **non-negotiables**: water, sunlight, sleep, movement, whole foods, quiet moments. These are your anchors.

A Note on Maintenance

Healing will change with each season. Some phases require more structure. Others need softness and rest. Check in with yourself like you would a close friend:

"How are you today? What do you need?"

Your body will answer.

Closing Reflection

You have learned to nourish, to listen, to slow down.
Now the invitation is to live — not carefully, but consciously.

Healing is not the absence of symptoms.
It is the presence of awareness, peace, and self-trust.

You are not returning to where you started.
You are moving forward — gently, wisely, at your own rhythm.

Every calm breath, every compassionate choice, every small pause is part of the path.

CHAPTER 19

SOS: ON THE DAYS WHEN NOTHING SEEMS TO BE WORKING

There will be days when inflammation returns, digestion feels reactive, hormones fluctuate, or fatigue becomes overwhelming — even when every effort toward healing has been consistent. These days are not evidence of failure. They are part of the biological rhythm of recovery.

Healing does not move in a straight line. It adapts to stress, sleep, environment, hormones, and nervous-system state. A flare occurs not because the body is breaking down, but because it is asking for support. Symptoms become communication rather than warning.

There were days I sat on the bathroom floor with a heating pad pressed against my stomach, nauseous, anxious, and exhausted. Pain like that makes you question your worth. I canceled plans, work assignments, trips — anything that required energy I didn't have. I watched opportunities slip away, along with people I once believed were friends.

What helped me most was learning to speak to myself the way I would speak to someone I love:
"This will pass. The discomfort is real, but so are you. You are stronger than this moment."

Sometimes even whispering those words felt like the only strength I had left, but it was enough to keep me soft instead of spiraling into fear.

UNDERSTANDING FLARE DAYS

A flare is a shift back into a protective mode. The nervous system perceives stress or instability, and the body responds by slowing digestion, increasing pain sensitivity, and conserving energy. These responses are not weaknesses. They are protective mechanisms that prioritize survival over repair.

On these days, the body is not asking for more effort. It is asking for gentleness.

THE SOS APPROACH: SIMPLIFY, OBSERVE, SUPPORT

Healing accelerates when the body is met with reduced pressure and increased safety.

Simplify

On flare days, remove excess demands. Avoid intense exercise, complicated meals, or large supplement combinations. Simplifying signals that there is no immediate danger and helps the nervous system return to equilibrium.

Observe

Noticing patterns brings clarity without blame. Sleep disruption, emotional stress, menstrual fluctuations, travel, overstimulation, skipped meals, or inflammatory foods can influence symptoms. Observation restores agency. Understanding a trigger is not punishment — it is knowledge.

Support

Warmth, hydration, rest, and easy digestion reduce the biological load. Support means choosing what brings stability rather than forcing productivity or "perfect" routines.

FLARE-FRIENDLY EATING

During a flare, the digestive system requires less stimulation and more warmth. Soups, broths, soft vegetables, warm grains, and gentle smoothies are easier to process than cold, raw, heavy, or highly seasoned meals. Warm herbal teas — such as ginger, chamomile, peppermint, or tulsi — calm both the gut and the nervous system. Nourishment becomes quiet rather than demanding.

PHYSICAL SOOTHERS

Simple physical interventions influence inflammation through the nervous system. Warm compresses and baths reduce muscular tension and increase blood flow. Magnesium absorbed through a warm bath can soften cramps and calm the stress response. Gentle stretching supports lymphatic flow, which helps remove inflammatory waste. Slow breathing lowers cortisol and reduces pain perception. These are physiological supports disguised as comfort.

EMOTIONAL CARE

Flares often evoke frustration, worry, or sadness. These emotions are natural responses to discomfort. Allowing expression — through writing, tears, or simply acknowledging difficulty — reduces internal pressure. Speaking to someone supportive releases oxytocin, a hormone that counteracts cortisol and decreases pain signaling. Even brief exposure to natural light can stabilize the circadian rhythm and soften irritability.

Sometimes the most healing thing you can do is admit, "Today is hard," and let that honesty be enough.

A DIFFERENT QUESTION

When symptoms arise, the habitual question becomes: *What did I do wrong?*
Yet a more accurate question is: *What does my body need today?*

Healing is not a search for perfection but a relationship with the body's signals. Each flare strengthens the capacity to return to balance. The skill is not to avoid every difficult day, but to respond without fear, urgency, or judgment.

A SIMPLE RESET

A flare day benefits from the same message expressed in multiple ways: reduce pressure, add warmth, preserve energy, and slow down stimulation. Limit screens, allow more rest, choose soft foods, and prioritize calm over productivity. These small adjustments reduce biological stress and shorten recovery time.

CLOSING REFLECTION

A flare is not a disruption of healing — it is a request for protection. The nervous system repairs itself through safety, not intensity. When discomfort is met with softness, the body exits survival mode more quickly and returns to balance with less effort.

On days when nothing seems to be working, your task is not to fix your body. It is to support it. The body heals most efficiently when it is no longer asked to fight.

PART V

THE 30-DAY RESET: A PRACTICE OF SAFETY & RESTORATION

CHAPTER 20

RETURNING TO YOURSELF

A healing plan is not a set of rules. It is an invitation to come back to your body. After years of reacting to symptoms, chasing answers, suppressing pain, or feeling betrayed by your biology, the Reset offers something much more powerful than control — it offers relationship.

You are not here to force your body into wellness. You are here to create the conditions in which wellness is possible.

For 30 days, you will eat, move, and rest in rhythm, giving your nervous system a reliable pattern it can trust. When the body feels safe, inflammation calms, digestion steadies, hormones regulate, and energy returns. This Reset is not about perfection. It is about practicing consistency without pressure — structure without strain.

Think of the next month as a season of repair. Every day does not need to be spectacular. It only needs to be supportive.

You are not fixing your body. You are learning how to care for it.

CHAPTER 21

WHAT THE RESET DOES

The Reset works by removing burden and offering nourishment. When inflammation is chronic, your biology becomes overwhelmed with signals — from stress, food, emotion, and environment. The reset quiets the noise so your body can hear itself again.

Over 30 days, you are giving your body:

- **Predictable rhythms** so cortisol can stabilize
- **Steady meals**, so blood sugar stays balanced
- **Warm, digestible foods**, so the gut can repair
- **Restorative movement**, so lymph and fascia can release inflammation
- **Daily calm**, so the nervous system stops bracing for danger

These practices settle inflammatory pathways, soften pain, reduce bloating, sharpen focus, improve sleep, and balance mood. Many women do not realize how good their body can feel until they stop demanding it to function under pressure.

The Reset is not restrictive—it is relieving.
It does not shrink your life. It expands your capacity to live in it.

CHAPTER 22

BEFORE YOU BEGIN: CREATE AN ENVIRONMENT OF HEALING

Healing improves most when your surroundings align with your goals. Before you begin, take a moment to prepare yourself and your space.

Prepare Your Mind

You are not trying to earn health through discipline. You are inviting health through respect. Your only job during the Reset is to listen to your body and respond with nourishment, gentleness, and rhythm. Some days will be energized, others quiet. This is normal. Biology does not move in straight lines — it moves in cycles.

Prepare Your Space

Create ease. Support your future self.

- Stock simple foods that can become warm meals: vegetables, legumes, quinoa, sweet potatoes, seeds, broths, herbs, teas, fresh fruit.
- Clear one shelf in your kitchen or fridge for reset foods.

- Make one corner of your home a calm space for breathing, journaling, or simply sitting without stimulation.

Healing thrives in predictability and simplicity. Complexity inflames; clarity restores.

Set Your Intention

Ask yourself:

- What do I want to feel more of?
- What am I ready to release?
- What does healing look like for me now?
- What kind of life do I want my body to support?

Your intention is not a goal to chase.
It is a direction to walk toward.

CHAPTER 23

THE FOUR ANCHORS OF THE RESET

The Reset rests on four daily practices. These are not rules, but anchors — quiet commitments that keep you connected to yourself.

1. Balanced Meals

Three meals a day. No perfection required. Each one includes:

- a source of fiber (vegetables, whole grains, fruit, legumes)
- a source of plant-based protein
- a source of healthy fat

Warmth matters. Digestion relaxes when food feels gentle.

2. Restorative Movement

Move daily — not to lose weight or "burn calories," but to circulate nutrients, reduce pain chemicals, and soften lymph congestion. Walk, stretch, do yoga, or practice Pilates. Twenty minutes is enough.

Your body does not need intensity to heal. It needs presence.

3. Sleep & Stillness

Go to bed with the intention of repair. Create dark, quiet evenings. Limit screens when the sun goes down. Rest during the day when your body asks. Stillness lowers cortisol more effectively than willpower.

4. Daily Calm

Stress is inflammatory. Calm is medicine. Even five minutes of breathwork, journaling, soft sound, warm tea, prayer, grounding, gentle touch, or silence signals safety to the body.

Healing is not the absence of stress. It is the practice of returning to calm.

CHAPTER 24

THE RESET IN PRACTICE

There is no perfect day on this Reset. There are only supportive days. A strong day is a day you nourish yourself. A strong day is a day you listen.

Morning

- Hydrate with water or herbal tea
- Have a warm breakfast rich in fiber, protein, and fats
- Step into natural light or take a quiet moment before screens

Afternoon

- Choose a warm, stabilizing lunch
- Move gently — a walk, stretching, or breathing
- Let your nervous system soften through slower eating and pauses

Evening

- Eat a light, calm dinner

- Reduce stimulants (screens, caffeine, loud environments)
- Let your mind unwind without demands or expectations
- Sleep early if possible — healing accelerates during deep rest

If you miss a day or feel overwhelmed, you do not start over. You simply begin again at the next meal or the next breath. Repair continues the moment you return to support.

CHAPTER 25

WHAT YOU WILL NOTICE

Healing is subtle at first. You might not wake up one morning suddenly pain-free. Change begins quietly:

- Digestion becomes calmer.
- Sleep deepens.
- Pain softens.
- Mood steadies.
- Cravings lessen.
- Energy feels more stable.
- Your body communicates more clearly.
- You respond more kindly.

Bloating may reduce. Anxiety may loosen its grip. Hormonal symptoms may feel lighter. You may feel less reactive to stress, food, and life. And gradually, something subtle begins to shift — not all at once, but in small ways that add up.

It took me a long time — years of trying, failing, and trying again — to understand what actually helped my body and what consistently triggered flare-ups. I had to learn how I reacted to stress, which products I needed to eliminate for good, and which ones became essentials I rely on every day. The real shift came quietly. One afternoon, I noticed that a situation which normally would have sent my body into a spiral… didn't. The discomfort stayed small, manageable, almost predictable. It sounds minor, but for me it was proof that something inside me was finally stabilizing. That moment made me want to share everything I had learned so other women wouldn't have to spend years guessing like I did. And yes — I still have my off-routine days. Healing didn't make me perfect; it simply means my body no longer punishes me the way it once did.

Most importantly, you begin to trust your body again — not because it never struggles, but because you now know how to support it. Healing is not the disappearance of symptoms. Healing is the return of connection.

AFTER THE 30 DAYS

WHAT COMES NEXT

The Reset may end today, but healing does not.

Your body has spent the last month remembering how to feel safe, nourished, and supported. Now the question becomes simple and profound:

How do you want to live with this new awareness?

What happens after the Reset is not a return to "normal," but a continuation of clarity. You have learned how your body responds to nourishment, rhythm, and calm. You have seen the difference between inflamed days and regulated days. You have experienced how much changes when you give your biology consistency instead of chaos.

The next chapter is about integration — choosing what stays.

Let the Reset Become a Reference Point

Your body is now speaking more clearly. You may notice signs you once ignored — slight bloating, subtle tension, shifts in mood, changes in sleep. These are not inconveniences; they are information.

Use what you learned this month to guide you, not restrict you. Ask gently, whenever symptoms arise:

"What is my body asking for?"

Sometimes the answer will be food.
Sometimes rest.
Sometimes boundaries.
Sometimes quiet.

Awareness is the real result of this Reset.

Choose What You Want to Keep

You do not need to hold onto everything. Choose only the practices that feel sustainable and supportive. The habits that grounded you, the meals that nourished you, the common-sense rhythms that made your body feel steadier — keep those.

Healing becomes effortless when you stop fighting your biology and start living with it.

Let Life Be Flexible

You will travel, eat out, work late, rush, celebrate, feel stressed, and have days that don't look like the last 30. This is not failure — it is life.

When things become chaotic, return to your anchors:

- a warm meal
- a slow breath
- ten minutes of quiet
- a walk outside
- an earlier bedtime

These small acts bring you back to balance more quickly now because your body remembers what balance feels like.

Expect Fluctuation, Not Perfection

Healing continues in layers. You may feel incredible for weeks and then have a difficult day. You may uncover new patterns, sensitivities, or strengths. This is not regression — it is integration.

Every flare you move through more gently is progress.
Every moment of awareness is progress.
Every time you choose support instead of pressure, your biology shifts.

You are no longer lost in your symptoms.
You understand their language.

Let Healing Move Into the Background

With time, this way of living becomes natural. You won't think about every meal, every feeling, every choice. You won't strive the way you did before. Healing moves from being a project to being a quiet rhythm supporting your life.

That is the real transformation.
Not the reset itself, but the relationship you build with your body because of it.

You Are Not Done – You Are Different

After 30 days, you do not return to who you were. You carry new awareness. New steadiness. A deeper sense of safety. A quieter nervous system. A clearer understanding of what helps you feel alive, balanced, and well.

The Reset is no longer something you follow.
It becomes something you live — gently, intuitively, with freedom and trust.

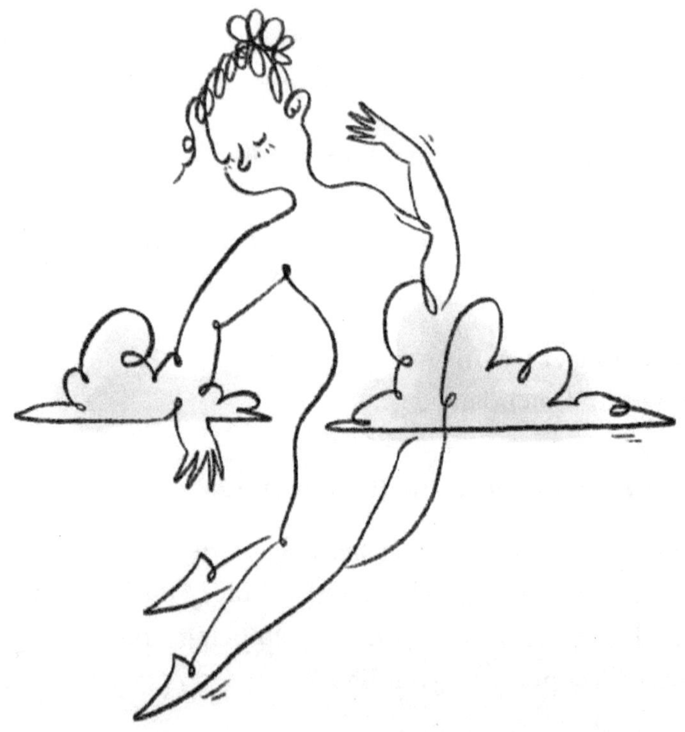

YOUR NEXT CHAPTER

Healing is not a final destination; it's an ongoing relationship with your body. By reaching this point in the book, you've already shifted something important — not because every symptom has disappeared, but because you now understand the difference between reacting to your body and partnering with it. You've learned how to recognize early signs of imbalance, how to respond with support rather than urgency, and how to return to calm more quickly than before. This knowledge is not abstract. It is lived, felt, practiced.

The next chapter of your life is not about rules or perfection. It is about remembering what your body has shown you: that it prefers rhythm to chaos, nourishment to restriction, warmth to pressure, and awareness to judgment. You now know which foods steady you, which routines help you feel grounded, and which choices invite inflammation or overwhelm. These insights are your compass. They guide without controlling, and they allow you to make decisions from clarity rather than fear.

There will still be difficult days. Every healing journey includes fluctuation — that is biology, not failure. What matters now is that you can meet those days differently. Instead of spiraling into worry, you can ask, "What does my body need today?" Instead of abandoning yourself, you can return to the practices that regulate your nervous system and ease inflammation. Healing becomes sustainable not because life becomes perfect, but because you have learned how to support yourself through imperfection.

As you move forward, choose what feels nourishing: meals that stabilize your energy, movement that strengthens without depleting, rest without guilt, boundaries that protect your peace, and environments — including people — that allow your nervous system to exhale. Let this way of living become part of your daily life, quietly guiding you in the background.

There will come a time when you notice that situations that once overwhelmed you now feel manageable. Your body will respond with less reactivity, your mind with more steadiness, and your energy with more consistency. That is not a dramatic transformation, but a real one — the result of cumulative softness, awareness, and support.

You are not returning to who you were before inflammation, stress, or chronic symptoms. You are moving into a more informed, connected version of yourself — someone who knows how to listen, how to respond, and how to trust her body again. This is your next chapter: not a protocol to follow, but a partnership to deepen. Healing does not disappear when the Reset ends. It evolves with you.

And now, you get to live in that new understanding — gently, confidently, and at your own rhythm.

APPENDIX A

FRUITS – HISTAMINE, FODMAP, AND ANTI-INFLAMMATORY GUIDE

Fruit	Histamine	FODMAP Sensitivity	Anti-Inflammatory Benefits	Comments
Blueberries	Low	Low	High in polyphenols; support gut & brain	Safe for daily use
Blackberries	Low–Moderate	Moderate	Anthocyanins reduce inflammation	Limit if bloating occurs
Raspberries	Low	Low–Moderate	Fiber supports microbiome diversity	Can ferment in IBS — use small portions
Strawberries	Moderate	Low	Rich in quercetin (mast cell support)	Avoid during histamine flare
Cranberries	Low	Low	Anti-inflammatory + urinary tract support	Best unsweetened
Dragon fruit (Pitaya)	Low	Low	Prebiotic fiber nourishes gut bacteria	Excellent for bloating
Physalis (Golden berries)	Low	Low	High vitamin C & carotenoids	Tart; good for immune support
Persimmon	Low	Low	Antioxidants & gut-calming tannins	Soothing in IBS; watch ripeness
Kiwi	Low	Low	Vitamin C + enzymes aid digestion	Excellent for constipation
Pineapple	Low	Moderate	Bromelain reduces pain + swelling	May irritate reflux
Papaya	Low	Low	Papain supports digestion	Great during flares
Banana (ripe)	Low	High	Supports serotonin pathways	Best ripe; limit if bloating
Banana (unripe/ green)	Low	Low	Resistant starch feeds microbiome	Great for gut healing; avoid if constipated

Mango	Low	High	High antioxidants + fiber	Try small portions for IBS
Watermelon	Low	High	Hydrating; high lycopene	Can trigger bloating in IBS
Apple	Low	High	Polyphenols support gut flora	Common trigger; test slowly
Pear	Low	High	Fiber supports motility	Can ferment in IBS; reintroduce slowly
Grapes	Low	Moderate	Resveratrol supports metabolic health	Best in small portions
Orange	Low	Low-Moderate	Vitamin C and hesperidin reduce inflammation	Avoid during reflux flare
Grapefruit	Low	Low	Anti-inflammatory flavonoids	Avoid with certain medications
Lemon / Lime	Low	Low	Digestive enzymes + vitamin C	Can irritate if stomach lining inflamed
Pomegranate	Low	Low	Potent antioxidant polyphenols	Excellent for endometriosis & PCOS
Cherries	Low	High	Melatonin supports sleep	Restrict if prone to bloating
Plum	Low	Moderate	Sorbitol supports bowel movement	May worsen diarrhea
Peach / Nectarine	Low	Moderate-High	Beta-carotene supports skin	Can irritate sensitive gut
Dates	Low	Low-Moderate	Supports beneficial bacteria	Best in small portions
Figs (fresh)	Low-Moderate	High	Polyphenols + minerals	Can trigger gas in IBS
Figs (dried)	High	High	High fiber + antioxidants	Avoid in histamine sensitivity

VEGETABLES – HISTAMINE • FODMAP • ANTI-INFLAMMATORY BENEFITS • NOTES

Vegetable	Histamine	FODMAP	Anti-Inflammatory Benefits	Notes / Comments
Zucchini	Low	Low	Gentle on gut; hydrating; easy to digest	Great during flares; cook lightly
Carrot	Low	Low	Beta-carotene supports hormone balance and skin repair	Best cooked for sensitive digestion
Pumpkin	Low	Low	Rich in antioxidants; calms gut inflammation	Avoid canned with additives
Sweet Potato	Low	Low	Stabilizes blood sugar and hormones	Japanese variety easiest for digestion
Bok Choy	Low	Low	Mild crucifer; supports estrogen detox	Least gas-forming crucifer

Spinach	Moderate	Low	Polyphenols reduce inflammation	Can trigger histamine symptoms
Kale	Moderate	Moderate	Flavonoids protect against inflammation	Steam; raw can stress digestion
Broccoli	Moderate	High	Sulforaphane aids hormone + liver detox	Introduce slowly; gas-forming
Cauliflower	High	High	Anti-inflammatory compounds	Common trigger in IBS + histamine
Cabbage	High	High	Supports detox + gut bacteria	Avoid when bloated; can ferment in gut
Bell Pepper	Low	Low	High vitamin C supports immune system	Red is sweetest and most nutrient-dense
Cucumber	Low	Low	Cooling + hydrating for gut lining	Peel if digestion is sensitive
Lettuce (all)	Low	Low	Gentle detox + hydration	Bibb/Romaine best for flares
Celery	Low	Low	Anti-inflammatory flavonoids	Supports hydration; good juice
Green Beans	Low	Low	Balanced fiber supports gut motility	Good cooked; avoid raw in flares
Asparagus	Moderate	High	Rich antioxidant profile	Can worsen gas/IBS
Eggplant	Moderate	Low	Nasunin protects cells	May trigger histamine in sensitive people
Tomato	High	Low	Lycopene reduces inflammation	Common histamine trigger; avoid in flares
Onion	Low	High	Quercetin reduces inflammation	Use infused oil for IBS
Garlic	Low	High	Natural antimicrobial + immune support	Best as oil for IBS; raw irritates gut
Mushrooms	High	Moderate	Beta-glucans support immunity	Histamine-releasing for many
Beetroot	Low	Moderate	Supports circulation + liver	Roast or boil to soften fibers
Radish	Low	Low	Detoxifying; stimulates bile flow	Can be spicy; juice is stronger
Arugula	Low	Low	Bitter greens aid hormone detox	Excellent raw; gentle on gut
Swiss Chard	Moderate	Low	High antioxidants; supports immunity	Can trigger histamine in some
Peas	Moderate	Moderate	Anti-inflammatory proteins	Introduce slowly if gassy
Corn	Moderate	High	Polyphenols support immune function	IBS trigger; avoid during flares
Potato (white)	Low	Low	Soothing starch; reduces gut stress	Best boiled or baked, not fried
Okra	Low	Low	Mucilage coats + heals gut lining	Excellent for reflux + IBS repair
Seaweed (nori, wakame)	Moderate	Low	Minerals support thyroid + immune health	Use small amounts; can release histamine

LEGUMES – HISTAMINE • FODMAP • ANTI-INFLAMMATORY BENEFITS • NOTES

Legume	Histamine	FODMAP	Anti-Inflammatory Benefits	Notes / Comments
Red Lentils (well-cooked)	Low	Low-Moderate	High polyphenols; steady plant protein	Best tolerated lentil during gut healing
Green / Brown Lentils	Moderate	Moderate	Fiber supports microbiome diversity	Must be well-cooked to reduce gas
Split Peas	Moderate	Moderate	Supports healthy blood sugar and satiety	Can cause bloating if undercooked
Chickpeas (cooked)	Moderate-High	High	Rich minerals support hormones + immunity	Hummus may be easier to digest
Chickpea Pasta	Moderate	High	Higher protein + fiber than wheat	Start with small servings
Black Beans	High	High	Anthocyanins support anti-inflammatory responses	Pressure cooking improves tolerance
Pinto Beans	High	High	Fiber reduces LDL and supports gut health	Best soaked + cooked slowly
Kidney Beans	High	High	Strong antioxidant activity	Must be fully cooked (toxin risk when undercooked)
White Beans	High	High	Resistant starch supports gut motility	Introduce slowly; gas-forming
Mung Beans	Low-Moderate	Low-Moderate	Cooling, anti-inflammatory in Ayurveda	Easier to digest than most beans
Soybeans (non-processed)	Low-Moderate	Moderate	Isoflavones support estrogen metabolism	Fermented forms higher histamine
Tempeh (fermented)	High	Low	Gut probiotics + anti-inflammatory proteins	Avoid in histamine issues
Natto (fermented)	High	Low	Contains vitamin K2 + enzymes	Hard to digest; not for IBS/histamine
Tofu	Low	Low	Gentle plant protein, cooling to digestion	Extra-firm easier to digest
Edamame	Moderate	Moderate	Rich in anti-inflammatory omega-6/omega-9	Can cause gas; eat in small portions
Pea Protein Powder	Moderate	Moderate	Clean protein alternative if additive-free	Can bloat if fortified or flavored

Important Note for Legumes

- ✓ Soaking + long cooking improves digestibility
- ✓ Pressure cooking reduces FODMAPs significantly
- ✓ Pureed forms (soups, spreads) are gentler for IBS
- ✓ Avoid cans with additives (gum, phosphates, citrates)
- ✓ Fermented legumes = high histamine, even if low FODMAP

GLUTEN-FREE GRAINS & STARCHES – HISTAMINE · FODMAP · ANTI-INFLAMMATORY BENEFITS · NOTES

Grain / Starch	Histamine	FODMAP	Anti-Inflammatory Benefits	Notes / Comments
Quinoa	Low	Low	Rich in magnesium + complete plant protein	Rinse well to remove bitter saponins
Brown Rice	Low	Low	Provides steady glucose + B vitamins	Soak if sensitive; easier digestion
White Rice	Low	Low	Gentle on gut; useful during flares	Not nutrient-dense; pair with veggies
Wild Rice	Low	Low	High in antioxidants + minerals	Chewier—best for strong digestion
Millet	Low	Low	Cooling grain; supports stomach + spleen	Good alternative for people with IBS
Buckwheat (not wheat)	Low	Low	Anti-inflammatory flavonoids (rutin)	Great for pancakes + porridges
Oats (gluten-free)	Low	Low-Moderate	Beta-glucans lower cholesterol + support gut lining	Avoid flavored or instant oats (additives)
Amaranth	Low	Low	Mineral-rich; supports bone + hormone health	Dense texture—cook thoroughly
Sorghum	Low	Low	Antioxidants + fiber for blood sugar stability	Works well as flour or cooked whole
Teff	Low	Low	Iron + calcium; nourishes energy + hormones	Basis of injera; warming grain
Sweet Potato	Low	Low	High in antioxidants + gut-supportive fiber	Best steamed or baked; avoid frying
Japanese Purple Sweet Potato	Low	Low	Anthocyanins reduce inflammation + support blood vessels	Excellent for skin + collagen support
Yucca (Cassava)	Low	Low	Resistant starch supports microbiome	Cassava flour still gentle — avoid overuse

Plantain	Low	Low	Supports stable blood sugar; prebiotic when green	Best baked, boiled, or air-fried
Potato (White/ Yellow)	Low	Low	Easy to digest + calming to nervous system	Avoid fried forms; bake/steam
Taro	Low	Low	Good for sensitive digestion; mineral-rich	Often tolerated when others aren't
Polenta (Cornmeal)	Low	Low–Moderate	Comforting grain that supports energy	Avoid GMO varieties; choose organic
Rice Noodles	Low	Low	Gentle substitute for wheat pasta	Avoid sauces with garlic/onion if IBS
Chickpea Pasta	Moderate	High	Higher protein; supports hormones	Watch for bloating; small portions
Cassava Flour / Tapioca	Low	Low	Supports gut as resistant starch when cooled	Use in rotation to avoid digestive heaviness

Quick Guidance

✓ Choose warm, cooked grains during gut healing
✓ Pair every grain with protein + fat to stabilize blood sugar
✓ Cooling grains (millet, white rice) work well during flares
✓ Warming grains (buckwheat, teff) support low metabolism & cold extremities

NUTS & SEEDS — HISTAMINE · FODMAP · ANTI-INFLAMMATORY BENEFITS · NOTES

Nuts / Seeds	Histamine	FODMAP	Anti-Inflammatory Benefits	Notes / Comments
Walnuts	Low	Low	Rich in ALA omega-3s; supports cardiovascular + brain health	Best raw/soaked; rancidity increases histamine
Almonds	Low	Low–Moderate	Vitamin E for skin + hormone support	Avoid large portions if IBS (limit 10–12/day)
Brazil Nuts	Low	Low	High selenium; supports thyroid + immunity	Limit 1–2/day to avoid excess selenium
Cashews	Moderate	High	Magnesium for nerves, muscles, mood	Often triggers bloating; avoid during flares
Pistachios	Low	Moderate	Lutein + antioxidants for eye/skin health	Limit handful; can worsen bloating in IBS
Pecans	Low	Low	Anti-inflammatory flavonoids + fiber	Heavy when roasted; raw/soaked best

Hazelnuts	Low	Low	Polyphenols support heart + skin barrier	Best in small portions to avoid gut heaviness
Macadamia Nuts	Low	Low	Heart-healthy monounsaturated fats	Very calorie-dense — small portions
Hemp Seeds	Low	Low	Complete protein + hormone support	Easy to digest; great for smoothies/salads
Pumpkin Seeds	Low	Low	Zinc + magnesium for hormones, immunity	Best lightly toasted or raw
Sunflower Seeds	Moderate	Low	Vitamin E + minerals; supports skin + mood	Can be inflammatory for some (seed oils allergy)
Sesame Seeds	Moderate	Low	Lignans support estrogen balance + liver	Can irritate IBS if large amounts
Flax Seeds	Low	Low	Omega-3s; supports bowel regularity + hormones	Must be freshly ground; drink water
Chia Seeds	Low	Low	Omega-3s; prebiotic gel supports gut lining	Must soak! Dry chia can cause bloating
Poppy Seeds	Low	Low	Good calcium + zinc for hormones	Use in small amounts; heavy in excess
Tahini (Sesame Paste)	Moderate	Low	Mineral-rich; supports skin + thyroid	Can be harder to digest; start small
Coconut (shredded, milk, butter)	Low	Low	MCTs = quick energy + antimicrobial effect	Can cause diarrhea in excess; start slowly
Nut/Seed Butters	Moderate	Varies	Concentrated vitamins + fats	Choose no-additives; portion 1–2 tbsp max
Pumpkin Seed Butter	Low	Low	High zinc for fertility + hormone balance	Good option if allergic to nuts
Almond Butter	Low	Low	Vitamin E + steady energy	Avoid flavored or sweetened versions

Quick Guidance

- ✓ **Soak nuts or eat raw to reduce histamine & improve digestion**
- ✓ **Avoid large portions — nuts are nutrient-dense and heavy**
- ✓ **Seeds are generally easier to digest than nuts**
- ✓ **During flares: choose hemp, chia (soaked), pumpkin, or soaked almonds**

HERBS & SPICES — HISTAMINE · FODMAP · ANTI-INFLAMMATORY BENEFITS · NOTES

Herb / Spice	Histamine	FODMAP	Anti-Inflammatory Benefits	Notes / Comments
Turmeric	Low	Low	Curcumin reduces inflammatory cytokines, supports liver + immune balance	Best with black pepper + fat for absorption
Ginger	Low	Low	Reduces nausea, supports gut motility, lowers cortisol	Ideal for IBS; tea is most soothing
Cinnamon (Ceylon)	Low	Low	Blood-sugar control + anti-microbial effect	Prefer Ceylon over Cassia (less toxic load)
Rosemary	Low	Low	Antioxidants protect brain + reduce oxidative stress	Can improve digestion if used lightly
Basil	Low	Low	Antioxidants, antimicrobial, supports gut microbiome	Fresh is better tolerated than dried
Parsley	Low	Low	Rich in vitamin C + supports detoxification	Helps reduce bloating from salt retention
Cilantro	Low	Low	Chelates heavy metals; antimicrobial	Can reduce gas + bloating for some
Oregano	Low-Moderate	Low	Antimicrobial, antifungal; powerful against gut pathogens	Strong — best used in small amounts
Thyme	Low	Low	Supports respiratory health + gut microbiome	Very strong; use small amounts in IBS
Mint (peppermint)	Low	Low	Relaxes digestive muscles, reduces IBS cramps	Tea is safest; raw leaves can trigger reflux
Dill	Low	Low	Soothes digestion, reduces gas	Great for IBS during flares
Fennel Seeds	Low	Low	Relieves bloating, supports gut motility	Excellent after meals as tea; avoid raw seeds in excess
Cumin	Low	Low	Aids digestion, reduces gas, increases enzyme secretion	Can be spicy for GERD; start small
Coriander Seeds	Low	Low	Improves digestion + balances gut bacteria	Often better tolerated than fresh cilantro
Paprika	Low-Moderate	Low	Mild antioxidants, supports circulation	Avoid spicy paprika if IBS or histamine flare
Black Pepper	Moderate	Low	Enhances absorption of curcumin; mild anti-inflammatory	Can trigger histamine in sensitive people

Chili / Cayenne	High	Low	Stimulates endorphins, circulation	Can cause flares: histamine, IBS, reflux
Cardamom	Low	Low	Calming digestive aid, supports liver enzymes	Good option for warm drinks + desserts
Cloves	Low	Low	Strong antimicrobial + numbing pain relief	Use small amounts due to potency
Garlic (fresh)	Low	**HIGH**	Anti-microbial, prebiotic, supports heart health	High FODMAP → avoid during IBS flares
Onion (fresh)	Low	**HIGH**	Antioxidants + prebiotic effects	High FODMAP → use infused oils instead
Onion/Garlic Oil	Low	Low	Keeps flavor without fermentable fibers	Best option for IBS or SIBO

Quick Guidance

✓ **Best for inflammation + IBS:** ginger, turmeric, fennel, dill, cilantro, cardamom

✓ **Use carefully if histamine-sensitive:** black pepper, paprika, oregano

✓ **Avoid during IBS flare:** garlic, onion *(use infused oils instead)*

✓ **For gas and bloating relief:** mint tea, fennel tea, cumin water, ginger

PLANT-BASED MILKS & YOGURTS – HISTAMINE • FODMAP • ANTI-INFLAMMATORY BENEFITS • NOTES

Product	**Histamine**	**FODMAP**	**Anti-Inflammatory Benefits**	**Notes / Comments**
Unsweetened Almond Milk	Low	Low	Vitamin E for skin + antioxidant support	Choose brands without gums or carrageenan
Almond Yogurt (plain, no gums)	Moderate	Low	Provides healthy fats + usable probiotics	Avoid added gums; choose low-histamine strains only
Coconut Milk (carton)	Low	Low	Supports hormone balance + nourishes gut lining	Avoid canned versions with BPA + thickeners
Coconut Yogurt (plain)	Moderate	Low	Best yogurt for low-histamine + gut repair	Choose brands with Bifidobacterium strains
Oat Milk (unsweetened)	Low	**Moderate**	Beta-glucans support gut + immune health	Higher carb → may spike glucose; choose no oils

Soy Milk (organic, unsweetened)	Low	**Moderate**	High protein, supports estrogen balance in small amounts	Avoid if thyroid issues + poorly tolerated in some IBS
Hemp Milk	Low	Low	Omega-3 fats + magnesium for nervous system	Great choice for histamine + IBS-friendly eating
Flax Milk	Low	Low	High lignans support hormone metabolism + estrogen clearance	Best for PCOS, endometriosis, acne
Cashew Milk	Low-Moderate	**Moderate**	Creamy texture + minerals (magnesium + zinc)	Can trigger bloating in sensitive IBS
Rice Milk	Low	Low	Easiest to digest, rarely causes reactions	High glycemic index → pair with protein/fat
Soy Yogurt (organic, plain)	Moderate	**Moderate**	Protein + probiotics can support gut in some	Avoid if histamine-sensitive or during IBS flare
Oat Yogurt (plain)	Moderate	**Moderate-High**	Prebiotic fibers support microbiome	Often contains gums + added sugars — read labels!
Coconut Kefir (no added sugar)	**High**	Low	Probiotic but can trigger histamine release	Avoid with histamine intolerance or flares

Low-Histamine Yogurt Probiotic Strains

✓ Safe & anti-inflammatory:

- *Bifidobacterium longum*
- *Bifidobacterium breve*
- *Bifidobacterium infantis* (now *B. animalis subsp. lactis*)
- *Lactobacillus rhamnosus GG*

✕ Avoid (histamine-producing strains):

- *Lactobacillus casei*
- *Lactobacillus bulgaricus*
- *Lactobacillus delbrueckii*
- Most kefir blends

Tip: Look for labels that list specific strains — if no strains are listed, skip it.

Quick Guidance

- ✓ **Best for histamine + IBS:** hemp milk, flax milk, coconut yogurt (with correct strains)
- ✓ **Use cautiously if histamine-sensitive:** almond yogurt, soy yogurt, oat yogurt
- ✓ **Avoid during flares:** any kefir (even coconut), high-FODMAP yogurts, flavored/sweetened plant yogurts
- ✓ **Gut-soothing pairings:** coconut yogurt + kiwi + chia, flax milk + cinnamon + blueberries

FERMENTED PLANT FOODS – HISTAMINE · FODMAP · ANTI-INFLAMMATORY BENEFITS · NOTES

Food	Histamine	FODMAP	Anti-Inflammatory Benefits	Notes / Comments
Sauerkraut (plain, unpasteurized)	**High**	Moderate	Beneficial Lactobacillus strains support immunity	Avoid during flares; can trigger histamine reactions
Kimchi (without fish sauce)	**High**	Moderate-High	Garlic + chili + probiotics reduce inflammation	Spicy + fermented = not histamine-friendly
Coconut Yogurt (plain)	Moderate	Low	Soothes gut lining + allows targeted probiotics	Choose **Bifidobacterium** + **L. rhamnosus** strains
Tempeh	**High**	Low-Moderate	Rich in protein + prebiotic fibers	Fermented soy → common histamine trigger
Miso Paste (gluten-free, white miso)	**High**	Moderate	Contains enzymes that support digestion	Avoid with histamine issues; use tiny amounts
Kombucha (unsweetened)	**High**	Moderate-High	Polyphenols + probiotics support microbiome diversity	Can worsen anxiety + flares due to histamine + caffeine
Pickles (naturally fermented)	**High**	Low-Moderate	Mineral-rich + supports microbiome if tolerated	Vinegar-free versions are better for gut, but still high histamine
Coconut Kefir	**High**	Low	Benefits gut bacteria diversity	Worst for histamine intolerance; avoid during flares
Gluten-Free Sourdough Starter (buckwheat or rice)	**Moderate-High**	Moderate	Partially digested grains = easier digestion	Still fermented → use only if no histamine symptoms

How to Use Fermented Foods Safely

✓ **Start small** — 1 teaspoon to 1 tablespoon + observe symptoms
✓ **Do not combine multiple fermented foods in a day**
✓ **Avoid during histamine or IBS flares**
✓ **Rotate instead of consuming daily**

Goal: microbiome diversity without overwhelming the immune system.

Low-Histamine Probiotic Strategy Without Fermentation

Instead of relying on fermented foods, support gut health with:

Method	**Benefit**
Specific probiotic supplements	Use targeted strains without histamine production
Prebiotic fibers (chia, flax, kiwi, cooked oats)	Feed beneficial microbes without fermentation risk
Polyphenols (berries, purple sweet potato, elderberry)	Act as "nutrition" for good gut bacteria
Aloe vera juice + ginger tea	Heal gut lining + reduce immune reactivity
Soaked chia pudding + kiwi	Excellent low-HIST low-FODMAP combination for microbiome growth

Best Probiotic Strains for Histamine & IBS

Choose:
Bifidobacterium longum
Bifidobacterium breve
Bifidobacterium infantis (B. lactis)
Lactobacillus rhamnosus GG

Avoid:
L. casei
L. bulgaricus
L. delbrueckii
Most kefir blends

Sweeteners, Sauces & Condiments

Item	Histamine	FODMAP	Anti-Inflammatory	Notes
Extra-Virgin Olive Oil (EVOO)	Low	Low	Strong	Rich in polyphenols; may reduce pain and inflammation; see detailed chapter.
Coconut Aminos	Low	Low–Mod	Moderate	Soy-free alternative to soy sauce; contains natural sugars, use in modest amounts.
Tamari (gluten-free)	Medium–High	Medium	Low–Mod	Can be high histamine due to fermentation; avoid during flares or high histamine periods.
Miso Paste	High	High	Moderate	Fermented; probiotic but high histamine. Use only if gut is calm and histamine tolerable.
Nutritional Yeast	Medium	Low	Low–Mod	Can trigger histamine in sensitive individuals; tolerable for some, inflammatory for others.
Mustard	Medium	Low	Low–Mod	Vinegar-based; avoid if vinegar triggers symptoms. Choose versions without artificial preservatives.
Apple Cider Vinegar	High	Low	Moderate	High histamine; avoid during flares; may aid digestion for some when tolerated.
Other Vinegars	High	Low	Low	Avoid with histamine issues. Can irritate acid reflux.
Tahini (sesame paste)	Low	Low–Mod	Moderate	Great for minerals and healthy fats; portion control for IBS.
Maple Syrup (pure)	Low	Low	Low–Mod	Best natural sweetener for sensitive digestion; use sparingly to avoid glucose spikes.
Coconut Sugar	Low	Low–Mod	Low–Mod	Lower glycemic than refined sugar; still a sugar — moderate use only.
Dates / Date Syrup	Low	Mod–High	Moderate	Great minerals and fiber; portion size matters for FODMAP.
Banana Puree (ripe)	Low	High	Low	Not ideal for IBS; use only in small amounts.
Monk Fruit (pure)	Low	Low	Low–Mod	Best no-glycemic impact option; avoid blended commercial mixes with additives.
Stevia (pure leaf or extract)	Low	Low	Low–Mod	Only pure versions; avoid blends using erythritol or maltodextrin.
Agave	Low	High	Low	High fructose, may worsen bloating and blood sugar. Use rarely.
Honey	High	High	Mod	High histamine and high fructose. Not recommended for histamine or IBS-sensitive bodies.

APPENDIX B

The Anti-Inflammatory Toolkit**
These tools do not replace medical care. They are daily, practical methods that reduce inflammation by calming the nervous system, improving circulation, and supporting gut repair. They work best when combined with stable nutrition, hydration, and restful sleep.

Healing is not instant. It's cumulative.
Small actions, repeated consistently, change biology.

1. RED LIGHT THERAPY (PHOTOBIOMODULATION)

For pain reduction, hormonal support, and tissue repair

What it does:
Red and near-infrared light penetrate the skin and reach the mitochondria—the energy factories inside cells. This light tells the mitochondria to produce more ATP (cellular fuel), which speeds healing and reduces inflammation.

Benefits supported in research include:

- reduced pain and menstrual cramps

- improved circulation and muscle relaxation
- support for thyroid and hormonal metabolism
- enhanced skin repair and collagen production
- improved mood and reduced fatigue

How to use it:

- Use 3–6 times per week.
- Keep 6–12 inches from the body (unless manufacturer states otherwise).
- Session length: 5–20 minutes depending on device size.
- Best timing: late afternoon or evening to relax the nervous system.
- Avoid directly over eyes and reproductive organs with high-power devices.

Where to use it on the body:

- lower abdomen/pelvis (for endo, cramps, IBS)
- thyroid/neck (short sessions only)
- face (for skin and mood)
- lower back (nervous system + organ support)

Who should be cautious:

- those with uncontrolled thyroid disorders should consult their doctor before shining light directly over the thyroid
- avoid use on active tumors
- avoid using immediately after strong exfoliants, retinoids, or photosensitizing medication

Why it works:
Red light reduces inflammatory cytokines, improves cellular oxygen use, and supports nitric oxide release—allowing tissues to relax

and receive more nutrients. It is a gentle, non-drastic therapy when used consistently.

2. MAGNESIUM FOR NERVOUS SYSTEM & PAIN RELIEF

Choosing the right type and timing

Magnesium is one of the most common deficiencies in women dealing with chronic inflammation, anxiety, endometriosis, PCOS, PMS, and insomnia. It regulates muscle tension, pain signaling, gut movement, blood sugar, and cortisol.

Not all forms are equal.

Best for Sleep, Anxiety, and Cramps

Magnesium Glycinate

- Relaxing
- Gentle on the gut
- Supports sleep and mood

Best for Constipation and IBS-C

Magnesium Citrate

- Pulls water into intestine, softens stool
- Use only if constipation is present
- Not ideal for those with loose stools

Best for Brain Fog, Mood & Focus

Magnesium Threonate (Mg-L-Threonate)

- Crosses the blood-brain barrier
- Helps with cognition, anxiety, and stress response

Best for Muscle Tension & Cramps (Topical)

Magnesium Chloride or Magnesium Sulfate (Epsom salt)

- Baths or sprays
- Good for people who cannot tolerate oral supplements

How to take it:

- Start low and increase gradually
- Best taken in the evening
- Avoid combining high doses with diarrhea, certain heart medications, or kidney disease

General starting range:
100–200 mg/night, gradually increasing to 300–400 mg/day if tolerated.
(Always consult a physician if on medications, especially for blood pressure or kidneys.)

Why magnesium matters:
Low magnesium keeps the nervous system in fight-or-flight mode. Balanced magnesium supports deep sleep, reduces prostaglandin activity (pain chemicals), lowers inflammation, and stabilizes blood sugar—making it foundational for healing.

3. VAGUS NERVE BREATHWORK

Switching your body from fight-or-flight to rest & repair

The vagus nerve runs from the brainstem through the face, lungs, heart, digestive organs, and reproductive system. It is the "brake" that slows stress hormones and allows digestion, hormones, immunity, and tissue repair to function.

When the vagus nerve is activated:

- digestion improves
- heart rate slows
- inflammation decreases
- cramps reduce
- sleep becomes deeper
- anxiety softens
- pain sensitivity lowers

The 4–7–8 Reset Breath

- Inhale through the nose for 4
- Hold gently for 7
- Exhale slowly through pursed lips for 8
  Duration: 3–5 minutes
  Best for: nighttime anxiety, IBS flares, cramps, tense days.

The "Humming Exhale"

- Inhale through nose
- Exhale with a low humming sound
  Why it works: the vibration directly stimulates the vagus nerve where it passes through the throat and chest.
  Benefits: anxiety reduction, improved digestion, emotional grounding.

The Body Scan + Breath

- Inhale, soften one area (jaw, shoulders, stomach)
- Exhale tension out
- Move down the body in segments
  This retrains your brain to interpret relaxation as safety.

Why this matters for inflammation:
Chronic stress turns on inflammatory cytokines even without injury. Breathwork lowers cortisol, reduces pain signaling, and rebalances immune responses.
With repetition, your baseline state shifts from survival to repair.

4. SOMATIC MICRO-RELEASE

Small movements that quiet pain and inflammation

When the body holds tension, fascia (the connective tissue surrounding muscles and organs) becomes tight and dehydrated. This traps inflammation, compresses nerves, and increases pain sensitivity. Micro-movement gently rehydrates fascia and sends "safety signals" to the brain, reducing pain.

These exercises are subtle, slow, and done without force.
They teach the nervous system to relax from the inside out.

Jaw + Diaphragm Release

For anxiety, headaches, pelvic pain, IBS flares

- Place the tip of your tongue on the roof of your mouth just behind the front teeth.
- Let the jaw drop open slightly without strain.
- Breathe slowly for 1–2 minutes.

Why it works: the jaw and diaphragm are neurologically linked. Relaxing one softens the other, reducing full-body tension.

Pelvic Drop Breath

For cramps, IBS, endometriosis, pelvic pain

- Sit or lie down comfortably.
- Inhale as if widening the hips from the inside.
- Exhale with a gentle sensation of dropping or melting downward.

This loosens pelvic floor guarding caused by pain and trauma.

Important:
Never force release. Tiny, supported shifts are more effective than stretching or pushing. Pain softens when the brain trusts the movement.

5. JOURNALING FOR NERVOUS SYSTEM SAFETY

Not venting — re-training the brain

Writing can heal, but **not all journaling is helpful.**
Venting repeatedly about stress or symptoms can keep the brain in survival mode by rehearsing danger.
Effective nervous-system journaling focuses on **safety and emotional processing, not re-living pain.**

The 3-Part Safety Journal

Use once daily or as needed.

1) What I'm experiencing:
Describe your physical or emotional state in 1–3 sentences.
Not a story, just facts.

"My stomach feels tight today and I'm overwhelmed."

2) What I know is true:
This step grounds the brain in reality.

"I've felt this before and it passes. My body is not in danger."

3) What I can offer my body right now:
List 1–2 supportive actions without pressure.

"I can breathe slowly and take a warm shower."

This shifts the nervous system from fear to support.
When practiced regularly, your brain begins to default to regulation instead of alarm.

6. DAO SUPPLEMENTS (SHORT-TERM HISTAMINE SUPPORT)

Useful temporarily, not a lifelong crutch

DAO (diamine oxidase) is the enzyme that breaks down histamine in the gut.
During periods of gut irritation, hormone shifts, or high stress, natural DAO production can drop.
A supplemental DAO enzyme can help prevent histamine spikes while deeper healing takes place.

When it may help

- reactions to fermented foods, alcohol, aged foods
- flushing, headaches, palpitations after meals
- new sensitivity during PMS or ovulation
- during travel or high-stress weeks
- IBS or histamine flare days

How to use

- Take immediately **before the first bite** of a meal that may trigger symptoms.
- Do not take on an empty stomach without food.
- Use for **temporary support**, not daily forever.

When to avoid

- If you are pregnant, breastfeeding, or have severe mast cell illness — consult a physician first.
- If you use it daily for months, it may be masking an underlying issue.
  In that case, focus on gut healing, stress regulation, and hormone balance.

DAO supplements help the body **while you restore your own capacity**.
They are training wheels, not a destination.

7. HERBAL NERVOUS SYSTEM SUPPORTS

Evidence-backed plants that calm without sedation

These herbs do not numb the nervous system — they support the biology of calm.

Tulsi (Holy Basil)

- Lowers cortisol
- Supports blood sugar balance
- Helps with anxiety and brain fog
- Mildly antimicrobial, supports gut health

Best as: tea, tincture, or capsule
Best time: morning or early afternoon
Avoid: during pregnancy without medical guidance

Chamomile

- Anti-inflammatory flavonoids calm gut and pelvic pain
- Mild muscle relaxant for cramps and headaches
- Promotes sleep and reduces anxiety

Best as: warm tea before bed or during flares
Avoid: if allergic to ragweed

Ginger

- Improves circulation
- Lowers nausea, cramps, and inflammation
- Enhances digestion and reduces pain sensitivity

Best as: grated ginger tea, broth, or added to meals
Caution: avoid in high amounts with blood-thinning medications

Why herbs matter biologically, not spiritually:
Plants contain adaptogens, polyphenols, and natural compounds that regulate the stress response, cortisol, gut motility, and pain signaling.
They do not force the body — they support its ability to balance.

10. GUT-LINING SUPPORT (FOOD-BASED, GENTLE REPAIR)

For bloating, acid flare, sensitivity, and IBS-type reactions

The gut lining renews itself every 2–6 days.
When inflammation, histamine, stress, or processed foods irritate it, the lining becomes more permeable ("leaky"), allowing immune cells to overreact to normal foods.
Repair does not require heavy supplements — simple soothing foods calm and rebuild the intestinal wall.

Warm Cooked Meals

The digestive system prefers warmth when irritated.
Heat relaxes the smooth muscles of the gut and supports enzyme activity, easing sensitivity and spasms.
Choose:

- warm oatmeal or quinoa
- cooked vegetables instead of raw salads
- blended soups and stews

Cold smoothies, raw bowls, and iced drinks can delay healing during flares.

Chia or Flax Gel

When soaked, these seeds form mucilage — a gel-like fiber that coats and soothes the intestinal lining.

How to use:

- soak 1 tablespoon chia or ground flax in warm water or plant milk
- let sit at least 10–15 minutes (or overnight)
- eat alone or add to warm breakfast or pudding

This supports bowel regularity, nourishes gut bacteria, and gently binds inflammatory byproducts.

Aloe Vera (Inner Gel Only)

Aloe vera contains acemannan, a polysaccharide studied for its ability to soothe and repair mucosal tissue. It acts like a cooling balm for an irritated digestive tract.

How to use:

- Use only the clear inner gel or juice labeled **inner fillet**
- Start with 1–2 teaspoons, increasing slowly to 1–2 tablespoons
- Best taken in the morning or before meals
- Avoid outer rind (latex), which can cause cramping or diarrhea

Aloe is particularly helpful during IBS flares, histamine reactions, heartburn, or after alcohol exposure.

Omega-3 Seeds (Chia, Flax, Hemp)

Omega-3s help rebuild the intestinal membrane and reduce inflammation. Omega-3 rich seeds support both the gut lining and hormonal balance.

Add 1–2 tablespoons daily to warm meals, puddings, or soups — consistency matters more than amount.

Chamomile Tea

Chamomile contains apigenin, a flavonoid that relaxes the gut's smooth muscles and reduces inflammation. Used at night, it supports digestion, mood, and sleep together.

Best during:

- periods of high stress
- sleep disruption
- menstrual cramps
- histamine spikes

This is not forever — it's a reset.
Once irritation calms, a wider variety of foods can be reintroduced comfortably.

SOUPS

1. VEGAN MINERAL BROTH

Ingredients:

- 2 carrots, chopped
- 2 celery stalks, chopped
- 1 zucchini, chopped
- 1 potato or sweet potato, chopped
- 1 small piece of kombu or wakame seaweed (optional, mineral boost)
- Handful fresh parsley
- 1 bay leaf
- 8 cups water

Method:

1. Add all ingredients to a large pot with water.
2. Bring to a boil, then simmer on low 1–2 hours.
3. Strain out vegetables (or blend for a gentle veggie soup).
4. Sip warm, season lightly with sea salt if tolerated.

2. CARROT & GINGER SOUP

Ingredients:

- 5 carrots, peeled + chopped
- 1 zucchini, chopped
- 1-inch piece of fresh ginger, peeled + grated
- 1 tbsp olive oil
- 4 cups vegetable broth (low sodium, onion/garlic free if sensitive)
- Salt to taste

Method:

1. In a pot, sauté carrots + zucchini briefly in olive oil.
2. Add ginger + broth, bring to boil.
3. Simmer until carrots are very soft (20–25 min).
4. Blend until smooth + creamy.

3. ZUCCHINI & POTATO PUREE SOUP

Ingredients:

- 3 medium zucchini, chopped
- 2 medium potatoes, peeled + diced
- 1 tbsp olive oil
- 1 tsp dried dill or parsley
- 4 cups water or mild veggie broth

Method:

1. Add zucchini + potatoes to pot with water/broth.
2. Simmer until potatoes are soft (20 min).
3. Blend until creamy, stir in olive oil + herbs.

4. BUTTERNUT SQUASH SOUP WITH TURMERIC

Ingredients:

- 1 butternut squash, peeled + cubed
- 1 carrot, chopped
- 1 tsp turmeric
- ½ tsp grated ginger
- 1 tbsp olive oil or coconut oil
- 4 cups water or broth

Method:

1. Roast or boil squash + carrot until tender.
2. Add to pot with ginger, turmeric, and broth.
3. Simmer 10 min.
4. Blend until silky.

5. RED LENTIL SOUP (VERY GENTLE)

Ingredients:

- 1 cup red lentils, rinsed well
- 1 carrot, diced
- 1 zucchini, diced
- 1 tsp cumin or turmeric (optional)
- 1 tbsp olive oil
- 5 cups water or broth

Method:

1. Place lentils, carrot, zucchini in pot with water/broth.
2. Bring to boil, then simmer until lentils fall apart (20–25 min).
3. Add olive oil, spices.
4. Blend if smoother texture is easier on digestion.

6. RICE & VEGGIE HEALING SOUP

Ingredients:

- ½ cup white rice (well rinsed)
- 1 carrot, chopped
- 1 zucchini, chopped
- 1 tbsp olive oil
- Pinch turmeric
- 5 cups water or broth

Method:

1. Add rice + veggies to pot with water/broth.
2. Simmer 30–35 min until rice is very soft.
3. Season gently, stir in olive oil.

✨ All of these soups are:

- **Vegan** 🌱
- Easy on the stomach (no raw cruciferous, no heavy spices)
- Can be pureed if smoother texture feels better

GENTLE VEGAN PEA SOUP

Ingredients:

- 1 cup **split peas** (or frozen green peas if split peas are harder to tolerate)
- 1 carrot, chopped
- 1 zucchini, chopped (optional, for lightness)
- 1 bay leaf
- 4–5 cups water or mild veggie broth (onion/garlic free if sensitive)
- 1 tbsp olive oil (add after cooking)
- Pinch of turmeric or cumin (optional, anti-inflammatory)
- Fresh parsley to garnish (optional)

Method:

1. Rinse peas well.
   - If using split peas: soak for 2–3 hours (helps digestibility).
2. Add peas, carrot, zucchini, bay leaf, and water/broth to a pot.
3. Bring to a boil, then simmer until peas are soft (split peas: ~40 min, green peas: ~15 min).
4. Remove bay leaf, blend until smooth.
5. Stir in olive oil before serving for creaminess.

DESSERTS

MILLET BERRY PUDDING

Ingredients (1 serving)

- ¼ cup dry millet (well rinsed)
- 1 cup water
- ½ cup unsweetened almond milk (or more for creaminess)
- 1 tsp vanilla extract or a pinch of cinnamon (optional)
- Fresh raspberries or other berries for topping
- Optional sweetener: ½ tsp maple syrup or stevia (if you want a touch of sweetness)

Instructions

1. Cook the millet: bring water to a boil, add millet, reduce heat to low, cover, and simmer until water is absorbed and millet is soft (≈20–25 min).
2. Let it cool slightly, then **blend in a Nutribullet** with almond milk until smooth and creamy.
3. Pour into a bowl or jar.
4. Top with fresh raspberries (or other berries), a sprinkle of cinnamon, or a few nuts/seeds if desired.
5. Enjoy warm or chilled—both work beautifully!

Notes & Variations

- Can add a tablespoon of Greek-style yogurt or vegan yogurt for extra creaminess and protein.
- For a chocolate version, add 1 tsp cacao powder while blending.
- Can be prepped ahead as **overnight millet pudding** for convenience.

CHOCOLATE CHERRY CHIA PUDDING

Ingredients:

- 3 Tbsp chia seeds
- ½ cup almond milk
- 1 tsp raw cacao powder
- ½ tsp vanilla extract
- ½ tsp maple syrup (optional)
- Fresh or frozen cherries for topping

Instructions:

1. Mix chia seeds, almond milk, cacao, vanilla, and sweetener.
2. Chill 2–3 hours or overnight.
3. Top with cherries just before serving.

SUNRISE GLOW BOWL

Servings: 1
Prep Time: 5–10 min (plus freezing time for turmeric/ginger cube)

Ingredients:

Frozen Turmeric/Ginger Cube:

- 1 tsp fresh grated turmeric
- 1 tsp fresh grated ginger
- 2–3 tsp coconut water or unsweetened plant milk
  (Blend and freeze in an ice cube tray beforehand)

Bowl Base:

- ½ cup frozen acai puree (unsweetened)
- ½ cup frozen dragon fruit chunks
- ½ cup plant-based protein smoothie (use pea protein or IBS-friendly powder)
- 2–3 Tbsp unsweetened plant milk to blend

Toppings:

- 1 Tbsp pumpkin seeds
- 1 tsp tahini (drizzle)
- Optional: a few fresh berries or edible flowers for extra visual appeal

FOODS FOR AN ANTI-INFLAMMATORY GLOW

(Plant-Based & Dairy-Free)

Introduction

Radiant skin is a reflection of inner balance. Chronic inflammation—often triggered by stress, processed foods, and environmental toxins—can manifest externally through acne, dullness, puffiness, and premature aging. Fortunately, food can be powerful medicine. By focusing on nutrient-dense, anti-inflammatory ingredients—especially those from the plant kingdom—you can nourish your skin, support hormonal harmony, and create a healthy glow from the inside out. This chapter explores the most potent skin-loving foods and how they contribute to long-term wellness and beauty.

1. Omega-3 Plant Power

Chia seeds, flaxseeds, hemp seeds, walnuts, seaweed

Omega-3 fatty acids are essential for calming inflammation and maintaining skin's moisture barrier. These fats help reduce redness, support hormonal balance, and improve skin elasticity. They also assist in maintaining supple, hydrated skin and reducing the appearance of fine lines. Seaweed adds additional anti-inflammatory compounds and is rich in iodine, which supports thyroid health—closely linked to skin clarity and energy.

2. Antioxidant-Rich Fruits & Vegetables

Berries, leafy greens, red cabbage, sweet potatoes, carrots, beets

These colorful powerhouses are loaded with antioxidants that combat free radicals, the unstable molecules that damage skin cells and accelerate aging. Berries are rich in vitamin C, which helps in collagen production. Leafy greens like spinach and kale provide vitamin A, which supports skin cell turnover. Sweet potatoes and carrots are high in beta-carotene, a precursor to vitamin A that helps protect skin from sun damage and keeps it glowing. Red cabbage and beets contain anthocyanins and betalains, which have strong anti-inflammatory and detoxifying effects.

3. Gut-Healing Fermented Foods

Sauerkraut, kimchi (vegan), coconut yogurt, miso

A balanced gut microbiome is crucial for skin health. Fermented foods introduce beneficial bacteria (probiotics) that help reduce systemic inflammation, improve digestion, and enhance nutrient absorption. When your gut is in harmony, the skin often reflects this with fewer breakouts, less redness, and a more even tone. Miso, made from fermented soybeans, is also rich in minerals like zinc, which supports wound healing and skin regeneration. Coconut yogurt provides probiotics without the inflammation potential of dairy.

4. Anti-Inflammatory Spices

Turmeric, ginger, cinnamon, cumin

Spices are concentrated sources of bioactive compounds with powerful anti-inflammatory properties. Curcumin, the active ingredient in turmeric, has been extensively studied for its ability to reduce inflammation at the cellular level. Ginger contains gingerol, which soothes the digestive system and reduces inflammatory markers in the body. Cinnamon helps regulate blood sugar, which in turn reduces inflammation and can prevent hormonal breakouts. These spices also support circulation, aiding in skin repair and detoxification.

5. Hydrating Plant Foods

Cucumber, watermelon, celery, romaine lettuce, herbal teas

Hydration is one of the most overlooked keys to skin luminosity. While drinking water is essential, eating hydrating foods ensures the body absorbs moisture more efficiently. Cucumber and watermelon are over 90% water and contain skin-soothing compounds like silica and lycopene. Celery supports liver function and helps flush out toxins. Herbal teas—especially nettle, hibiscus, and chamomile—are rich in antioxidants and help reduce bloating, which can dull the skin's appearance.

6. Skin-Loving Healthy Fats

Avocados, olive oil, almonds, pumpkin seeds, tahini

Healthy fats are vital for maintaining the lipid barrier of the skin, which protects against moisture loss and external irritants. Avocados provide vitamin E, a powerful antioxidant that neutralizes free radicals and supports skin repair. Olive oil, particularly extra virgin, contains polyphenols and squalene, which combat oxidative stress and smooth skin texture. Pumpkin seeds are rich in zinc and magnesium, two minerals important for hormonal balance and inflammation control. Tahini, made from sesame seeds, is high in lignans and healthy fats that support detoxification pathways and skin regeneration.

7. Medicinal & Adaptogenic Mushrooms

Shiitake, maitake, lion's mane, reishi, chaga, king trumpet

Mushrooms are unique in their ability to modulate the immune system and reduce chronic inflammation. Shiitake mushrooms contain kojic acid, which supports collagen production and can brighten uneven skin tone. Reishi and chaga are adaptogens that help the body cope with stress—a major internal cause of skin issues. Lion's mane supports gut health and brain function, contributing to reduced stress-related inflammation. King trumpet mushrooms are especially high in antioxidants like ergothioneine, which protects cells from oxidative damage and supports tissue repair. Their meaty texture also makes them a perfect whole-food alternative to processed meat replacements.

8. Purple Power: Anti-Aging Vegetables

Eggplant, Japanese sweet potato, purple carrots, purple cabbage, purple cauliflower

Purple vegetables owe their vibrant hue to **anthocyanins**, powerful antioxidants that protect cells from oxidative stress and slow down visible signs of aging. These pigments help increase blood flow, support collagen maintenance, and reduce skin inflammation. Japanese purple sweet potatoes are rich in complex carbohydrates, fiber, and vitamin C—helping to stabilize blood sugar and fuel the skin's regenerative processes. Eggplants contain nasunin, a unique antioxidant that protects the skin's lipid membranes and may guard against UV damage. Purple carrots and cauliflower offer a spectrum of phytonutrients that defend against premature aging while supporting a youthful glow.

ANTI-INFLAMMATORY GLOW JUICE
(3–4 SERVINGS)

Ingredients:

- 19 stalks of celery
- 6 boiled beetroots (medium)
- 2 whole pieces of fresh ginger (peeled)
- 2 whole pieces of fresh turmeric (peeled)
- 4 apples (medium)
- 1 cup pineapple (fresh or frozen)

Instructions:

1. Juice the celery first, followed by apples and pineapple for a sweet base.
2. Add the boiled beets to mellow out the earthiness and boost circulation.
3. Finish with ginger and turmeric for a powerful anti-inflammatory and antioxidant punch.
4. Stir well and store in glass bottles or jars. Keep refrigerated and consume within 4 days.

Why it works:

This juice is rich in betalains from beets (which support detox and reduce inflammation), bromelain from pineapple (a natural anti-inflammatory enzyme), polyphenols from apples, and powerful compounds like curcumin and gingerol. Celery hydrates and supports digestion, making this a skin-clearing, energy-boosting tonic you'll want to sip daily.

THE POWER OF A VIRGIN OLIVE OIL SHOT

Liquid gold for your skin, hormones, and longevity

A daily **shot of high-quality extra virgin olive oil** (about 1 tablespoon) is one of the simplest yet most powerful rituals for reducing inflammation, supporting cellular health, and nurturing radiant skin from the inside out.

🌿 Top Benefits of Olive Oil Shots:

1. Anti-Inflammatory Hero
Extra virgin olive oil (EVOO) is rich in *oleocanthal*, a natural compound that works similarly to ibuprofen—without the side effects. It reduces systemic inflammation, easing everything from puffiness to joint stiffness and inflammatory skin conditions like acne, rosacea, and eczema.

2. Hormone Support
Healthy fats are essential for hormone production and balance, especially estrogen and progesterone. A daily olive oil shot nourishes the endocrine system and supports smoother menstrual cycles, better mood stability, and glowing skin.

3. Gut & Liver Love
Olive oil acts as a gentle stimulant for bile flow and digestion, supporting liver detoxification—key for clear skin and energy. It also improves nutrient absorption, especially for fat-soluble vitamins like A, D, E, and K.

4. Antioxidant-Rich Glow
Packed with polyphenols, EVOO protects your skin from oxidative stress and free radical damage—the main culprits behind premature aging. Regular intake can improve skin texture, reduce fine lines, and enhance that natural, lit-from-within look.

5. Cardiovascular & Brain Health

Olive oil's monounsaturated fats help reduce LDL ("bad") cholesterol while increasing HDL ("good") cholesterol. It also supports brain function, memory, and mood—making it a beauty ritual that benefits mind and body alike.

Why the Quality of Olive Oil Matters

Unfortunately, not all olive oil is created equal. Many brands on supermarket shelves are **blended, oxidized, or even cut with cheaper seed oils**, reducing their health benefits and increasing inflammation instead of reducing it.

🕵 How to Choose Real Extra Virgin Olive Oil:

- **Look for cold-pressed or first cold-pressed:** This ensures minimal processing and higher nutrient content.
- **Check for harvest or press date:** Use within 18 months of harvest for maximum benefits.
- **Choose dark glass bottles:** Protects the oil from light damage.
- **Avoid "light" or "pure" olive oil:** These are refined and stripped of most nutrients.
- **Taste it:** Good EVOO should taste peppery, slightly bitter, and grassy—those are the polyphenols at work.

How to Take It:

- **Morning Ritual:** 1 tbsp on an empty stomach, optionally with a squeeze of lemon.
- **Pre-Meal Booster:** Take it 15 minutes before meals to stimulate digestion and enhance fullness.
- **Skin Glow Shot:** Combine with a pinch of turmeric and black pepper for enhanced anti-inflammatory action.

MATCHA MAGIC

A calm, clean energy + antioxidant powerhouse

Matcha is a finely ground powder made from specially grown and processed green tea leaves. Unlike traditional green tea where you steep and discard the leaves, with matcha, you consume the **entire leaf**—which means you're getting a **mega-dose of nutrients, chlorophyll, and antioxidants**.

🍵 Glow Benefits of Matcha:

1. Packed with EGCG: A Skin-Saving Antioxidant
Matcha is especially rich in **EGCG (epigallocatechin gallate)**, one of the most powerful antioxidants known to science. EGCG helps combat free radicals, reduce UV damage, and protect collagen—making your skin more resilient, firm, and clear.

2. Calms Inflammation from the Inside Out
Matcha is a natural anti-inflammatory, helping to reduce redness, puffiness, and inflammatory skin conditions like acne and eczema. It also helps regulate sebum production, keeping pores clearer.

3. Supports Detox + Liver Function
Thanks to its high chlorophyll content, matcha helps cleanse the blood and liver. A clean liver = clearer skin and more hormonal harmony.

4. Natural Energy Without the Crash
Matcha contains caffeine, but it's paired with **L-theanine**, an amino acid that promotes calm focus and balanced energy. No jitters, no crash—just steady alertness that helps keep cortisol (your stress hormone) in check.

5. Gut + Microbiome Support

Green tea polyphenols have been shown to support a healthy microbiome and reduce "bad" bacteria while feeding the good ones. A happy gut = glowing skin.

PEAS: THE PLANT-BASED PROTEIN WITH GLOW BENEFITS

Whether fresh, frozen, or powdered into protein, **green peas** are a fantastic vegan protein source—and they bring a lot more to the table than just muscle support.

Protein Content:

- **9g of protein per cooked cup**
- Rich in **essential amino acids**, especially lysine (great for skin + collagen repair)
- Often used as the base for **vegan protein powders** because of their digestibility

Why Peas Are Glow-Friendly:

1. Skin-Nourishing Micronutrients

Peas are rich in **vitamin C**, **vitamin A**, and **vitamin K**—all of which help support collagen production, reduce inflammation, and promote skin healing.

2. Hormone-Balancing Fiber

They're packed with **soluble fiber**, which helps regulate blood sugar and supports estrogen detox through the gut—key for hormonal acne and PMS support.

3. Gut-Loving + Easy on Digestion
Unlike some legumes, peas are relatively gentle on the digestive system, especially when cooked. A healthy gut = better nutrient absorption + clearer skin.

4. Low in Fat, High in Nutrients
They're a great addition if you're balancing hormone-supportive fats from other sources (like seeds and olive oil), and still want that protein boost.

Lifestyle & Stress Reduction

Skincare from the Inside Out

Success Stories & Testimonials

DAILY DRY BRUSHING

A 5-minute ritual for detox, circulation, and glowing skin

Dry brushing is an ancient Ayurvedic self-care practice that stimulates the **lymphatic system**, boosts **circulation**, and gently exfoliates the skin. Just a few minutes a day can leave your skin noticeably smoother and help your body eliminate toxins more efficiently.

Glow Benefits of Dry Brushing:

1. Boosts Circulation
The brushing motion increases blood flow, which delivers oxygen and nutrients to your skin cells—leading to a fresh, radiant complexion and natural color.

2. Lymphatic Drainage

Dry brushing stimulates the lymphatic system, helping your body flush out waste, reduce bloating, and support immune health. A sluggish lymph system can contribute to dullness, acne, and water retention.

3. Natural Exfoliation

It removes dead skin cells and unclogs pores, improving skin texture and allowing moisturizers or body oils to absorb more effectively.

4. Supports Cell Renewal & Collagen Production

Regular stimulation encourages cell turnover and collagen synthesis, helping reduce the appearance of cellulite and improving skin tone and elasticity.

How to Dry Brush Properly:

1. Use a **natural bristle brush** (not synthetic).
2. Always brush **toward your heart**—start from your feet and move upward in long, sweeping motions.
3. Use light to medium pressure. The goal is stimulation, not irritation.
4. Focus on areas where lymph nodes are concentrated: behind knees, underarms, inner thighs.
5. Follow with a shower and apply a nourishing body oil (like olive oil, sesame oil, or jojoba).

Tip: For added benefits, do your dry brushing before a sauna or after applying a body serum for enhanced absorption.

SIMPLE DAILY RESET ROUTINE (EXAMPLE)

This routine is intended as an example of how supportive daily habits may be structured to promote nervous system balance, hormone regulation, and overall well-being. It can be adapted based on individual needs, energy levels, and lifestyle.

Morning (5–60 minutes, depending on availability)

- a glass of water (optionally with lemon or minerals)
- light movement or a longer session such as Pilates or gentle exercise
- brief breathing practice or meditation
- writing down three things you are grateful for to support emotional balance

During the day

- balanced meals that include protein, fiber, and healthy fats
- paying attention to adequate protein intake throughout the day
- incorporating fiber-rich foods to support digestion and elimination

- including probiotic foods such as sauerkraut or vegan yogurt with added probiotics
- gentle movement such as walking
- consistent hydration throughout the day
- social connection, such as meeting a friend or speaking with a loved one
- if your day involves prolonged sitting, taking short breaks every hour to stand, stretch, or walk can support circulation and reduce physical tension, stiffness, and discomfort

Evening (10–20 minutes)

- reduce screen exposure
- calming activity such as journaling, reading, or light stretching
- optional relaxation practice such as meditation or tapping

This routine is not meant to be followed perfectly. Even small, consistent actions can support regulation and recovery over time.

MEDICAL GLOSSARY

Adaptogens

Natural plant compounds that help the body regulate its response to stress. Adaptogens support balance within the nervous system and stress hormones such as cortisol. Rather than stimulating or sedating directly, they promote resilience and recovery over time.

Autoimmune Disease

A condition in which the immune system mistakenly attacks the body's own tissues. Chronic inflammation and immune dysregulation are central mechanisms in autoimmune disorders.

Blood Sugar Regulation

The body's ability to maintain stable glucose levels in the bloodstream. Balanced blood sugar supports stable energy, mood, and hormonal health, while repeated spikes and crashes can contribute to inflammation and metabolic stress.

Circadian Rhythm

The body's internal 24-hour biological clock that regulates sleep, hormone release, metabolism, digestion, and immune function.

Disruption of circadian rhythm—through late nights, artificial light, or irregular routines—can increase inflammation and hormonal imbalance.

Chronic Inflammation

Low-grade, persistent immune activation that lasts for months or years. Unlike acute inflammation, it often has no obvious symptoms at first, yet it plays a central role in many modern conditions, including autoimmune disorders and metabolic dysfunction.

Cortisol

A stress hormone produced by the adrenal glands. It helps regulate blood sugar, blood pressure, and the body's response to stress. Chronically elevated or dysregulated cortisol can disrupt sleep, increase inflammation, and interfere with hormonal balance.

Cytokines

Signaling proteins released by immune cells. They help coordinate the body's inflammatory response. When overproduced, cytokines can drive chronic inflammation and tissue damage.

Dysbiosis

An imbalance in the gut microbiome in which harmful bacteria or yeast outnumber beneficial microbes. Dysbiosis can contribute to inflammation, digestive symptoms, hormonal disruption, immune dysfunction, and mood instability.

Dysregulation

A disruption in the body's normal regulatory systems. When biological systems such as the immune system, hormones, metabolism, or the nervous system become dysregulated, they may function either excessively or insufficiently. Chronic dysregulation can contribute to persistent inflammation, metabolic disturbances, hormonal imbalance, and increased vulnerability to disease.

Endocrine Disruptors

Chemical compounds that interfere with the body's hormonal signaling. These substances may mimic, block, or alter natural hormones such as estrogen, progesterone, thyroid hormones, insulin, and cortisol. Chronic exposure can increase inflammation and contribute to hormone-related conditions.

Estrogen

A primary female sex hormone involved in reproductive health, bone density, brain function, and cardiovascular protection. Balanced estrogen levels are essential for overall hormonal stability.

Estrogen Dominance

A state in which estrogen activity outweighs progesterone activity, either due to excess estrogen, low progesterone, or impaired estrogen detoxification. This imbalance may intensify inflammation, menstrual pain, fluid retention, mood swings, and other hormone-related symptoms.

Gut-Brain Axis

The gut–brain axis refers to the bidirectional communication network between the gastrointestinal system and the central nervous system. This connection involves neural pathways, hormones, immune signals, and microbial metabolites produced by the gut microbiome. Disruptions in this communication may influence digestion, mood, inflammation, and stress responses.

Gut Microbiome

The complex ecosystem of microorganisms living in the digestive tract, including bacteria, fungi, viruses, and other microbes. A balanced microbiome supports immunity, nutrient absorption, hormonal regulation, and mental health. Disruption may contribute to inflammation and chronic symptoms.

Histamine

A chemical messenger involved in immune responses, digestion, and nervous system signaling. While histamine plays protective roles, excessive levels or reduced breakdown can contribute to inflammation, headaches, skin reactions, anxiety, and digestive symptoms.

Hormonal Imbalance

A disruption in the normal relationship between hormones such as estrogen, progesterone, insulin, cortisol, and thyroid hormones. Even small imbalances can affect mood, metabolism, sleep, and inflammatory responses.

Inflammation

A natural defense response of the immune system. In the short term, it protects the body from injury and infection. When it becomes chronic, it can quietly damage tissues and contribute to pain, fatigue, hormonal imbalance, and long-term disease.

Insulin

A hormone produced by the pancreas that allows cells to absorb glucose from the bloodstream for energy. Proper insulin function is essential for stable energy levels and metabolic health.

Insulin Resistance

A condition in which cells become less responsive to insulin, the hormone responsible for regulating blood sugar. Over time, this can lead to elevated glucose levels, increased fat storage, energy instability, and a higher risk of metabolic disease.

Intestinal Permeability ("Leaky Gut")

A condition in which the intestinal barrier becomes compromised, allowing unwanted particles to pass into the bloodstream. This may trigger immune activation and contribute to systemic inflammation.

Irritable Bowel Syndrome (IBS)

A functional gastrointestinal disorder characterized by abdominal pain, bloating, and altered bowel habits (constipation, diarrhea, or both) without visible structural damage to the intestines. While IBS is not classified as an inflammatory bowel disease, low-grade inflammation, gut–brain axis dysregulation, microbiome imbalance, and stress-related nervous system activation often contribute to symptoms.

Lymphatic System

A network of vessels and nodes responsible for clearing waste, toxins, excess fluid, and inflammatory molecules from tissues. Unlike the circulatory system, it relies on movement, breathing, and muscle contraction to function efficiently. Stagnation may contribute to swelling, fatigue, and persistent inflammation.

Metabolism

Metabolism refers to the complex network of chemical processes that occur in the body to maintain life. These processes convert nutrients from food into energy, build and repair tissues, and regulate essential functions such as hormone activity, temperature control, and cellular maintenance. Metabolism includes two main types of reactions: catabolism, which breaks down molecules to release energy, and anabolism, which uses energy to build and repair cells and tissues.

Metabolic Dysfunction

Metabolic dysfunction refers to impaired regulation of the body's energy systems, including abnormalities in glucose metabolism, insulin signaling, fat storage, and mitochondrial energy production. Over time, metabolic dysfunction may contribute to chronic inflammation, insulin resistance, fatigue, and increased risk of metabolic and cardiovascular disease.

Microbiome

The microbiome refers to the collective genetic material of all microorganisms living in a specific environment, such as the human gut, skin, or mouth. In the context of human health, the gut microbiome plays an important role in digestion, immune system regulation, metabolism, and the production of certain vitamins and signaling molecules.

Microbiota

Microbiota refers to the community of microorganisms—such as bacteria, viruses, fungi, and other microbes—that live in a specific environment of the body, most notably the gastrointestinal tract.

These microorganisms interact with the immune system, influence digestion, and contribute to metabolic and physiological processes important for overall health.

Mitochondria

Structures within cells responsible for producing energy in the form of ATP. Often described as the "power plants" of the cell, healthy mitochondria are essential for metabolism, hormonal balance, and overall vitality.

Nervous System Regulation

The balance between the sympathetic ("fight or flight") and parasympathetic ("rest and repair") branches of the nervous system. Long-term stress dominance can sustain inflammation and disrupt hormonal health.

Oxidative Stress

A physiological state in which the production of reactive oxygen species (free radicals) exceeds the body's antioxidant defenses. While small amounts are necessary for normal cellular signaling, chronic excess damages lipids, proteins, and DNA, impairing mitochondrial function and amplifying inflammation.

Progesterone

A hormone that supports menstrual cycle regulation, fertility, and nervous system balance. Adequate progesterone helps counterbalance estrogen and promotes calm, restorative processes in the body.

Prostaglandins

Hormone-like compounds involved in inflammation, pain signaling, and uterine contractions. Certain prostaglandins increase inflammatory responses and are associated with menstrual pain and inflammatory conditions.

Thyroid Hormones

Hormones produced by the thyroid gland that regulate metabolism, temperature, energy production, digestion, and mood. Imbalances can contribute to fatigue, weight changes, hormonal instability, and inflammatory patterns.

Zonulin

A protein that regulates the permeability of the intestinal lining. Elevated zonulin levels are associated with increased intestinal permeability ("leaky gut"), which may trigger immune activation and systemic inflammation.

REFERENCES

AbbVie. (2022). *Global Gastrointestinal Health Survey.* AbbVie Inc.

Barnett, M. P. G., McNabb, W. C., Roy, N. C., Woodford, K. B., & Clarke, A. J. (2015). A1 β-casein: Impact on gastrointestinal function and inflammation. *Nutrition Journal,* 14, 38.

Belkaid, Y., & Hand, T. W. (2014). Role of the microbiota in immunity and inflammation. *Cell,* 157(1), 121–141.

Boberg, J., Taxvig, C., Christiansen, S., & Hass, U. (2010). Possible endocrine disrupting effects of parabens and their metabolites. *Critical Reviews in Toxicology,* 40(7), 622–632.

Carabotti, M., Scirocco, A., Maselli, M. A., & Severi, C. (2015). The gut–brain axis: Interactions between enteric microbiota, central and enteric nervous systems. *Annals of Gastroenterology,* 28(2), 203–209.

De Filippis, F., Vitaglione, P., Cuomo, R., Berni Canani, R., & Ercolini, D. (2018). Diet, environment, and the gut microbiome. *Nature Reviews Gastroenterology & Hepatology,* 15(2), 109–120.

Endocrine Society. (2015). Endocrine-disrupting chemicals: An Endocrine Society scientific statement. *Endocrine Reviews,* 36(6), E1–E150.

Fasano, A. (2012). Zonulin, regulation of tight junctions, and autoimmune diseases. *Annals of the New York Academy of Sciences,* 1258, 25–33.

Furman, D., Campisi, J., Verdin, E., et al. (2019). Chronic inflammation in the etiology of disease across the life span. *Nature Medicine,* 25(12), 1822–1832.

Harvard T.H. Chan School of Public Health. (n.d.). *Inflammation and diet.* Harvard University.

Hayes, T. B., et al. (2011). Atrazine induces complete feminization and chemical castration in male African clawed frogs. *Journal of Steroid Biochemistry and Molecular Biology,* 127(1–2), 64–73.

Hemarajata, P., & Versalovic, J. (2013). Effects of probiotics on gut microbiota: Mechanisms of intestinal immunomodulation. *Therapeutic Advances in Gastroenterology,* 6(1), 39–51.

Iliev, I. D., & Leonardi, I. (2017). Fungal dysbiosis: Immunity and interactions at mucosal barriers. *Nature Reviews Immunology,* 17(10), 635–646.

Leslie, H. A., et al. (2022). Discovery and quantification of plastic particles in human blood. *Environment International,* 163, 107199.

Lu, G. D., & Needham, J. (2004). *Celestial Lancets: A History and Rationale of Acupuncture and Moxa.* Routledge.

Maintz, L., & Novak, N. (2007). Histamine and histamine intolerance. *American Journal of Clinical Nutrition,* 85(5), 1185–1196.

Medzhitov, R. (2008). Origin and physiological roles of inflammation. *Nature,* 454(7203), 428–435.

Meeker, J. D., Sathyanarayana, S., & Swan, S. H. (2009). Phthalates and other additives in plastics: Human exposure and associated health outcomes. *Human Reproduction Update,* 15(3), 253–265.

Melnik, B. C. (2011). Milk consumption: Aggravating factor of acne and promoter of chronic diseases of Western societies. *Journal of Dermatological Science,* 64(3), 179–186.

Maté, G. (2003). *When the Body Says No: The Cost of Hidden Stress.* Vintage Canada.

Maté, G. (2022). *The Myth of Normal: Trauma, Illness & Healing in a Toxic Culture.* Knopf Canada.

Olszewski, W. L. (2003). Lymphatic system in body homeostasis: Physiological conditions. *Lymphatic Research and Biology,* 1(1), 11–21.

Peretz, J., et al. (2014). Bisphenol A and reproductive health: Update of experimental and human evidence. *Reproductive Toxicology,* 50, 1–13.

Randolph, G. J., Ivanov, S., Zinselmeyer, B. H., & Scallan, J. P. (2017). The lymphatic system: Integral roles in immunity. *Annual Review of Immunology,* 35, 31–52.

Rea, K., Dinan, T. G., & Cryan, J. F. (2021). The microbiome: A key regulator of stress and neuroinflammation. *Neurobiology of Stress,* 15, 100352.

Rier, S. E., et al. (2001). Endometriosis in rhesus monkeys exposed to dioxin. *Toxicological Sciences,* 59(1), 147–159.

Round, J. L., & Mazmanian, S. K. (2009). The gut microbiota shapes intestinal immune responses. *Nature Reviews Immunology,* 9(5), 313–323.

Schwingshackl, L., et al. (2021). Adherence to Mediterranean diet and inflammatory markers. *Nutrients,* 13(5), 1514.

Sharma, P. V., & Dash, B. (2017). *Charaka Samhita: Text with English Translation.* Chowkhamba Sanskrit Series.

Sims, S. (2016). *ROAR: How to Match Your Food and Fitness to Your Unique Female Physiology.* Rodale.

Sperber, A. D., et al. (2021). Worldwide prevalence and burden of functional gastrointestinal disorders. *Gastroenterology,* 160(1), 99–114.

Steinemann, A., et al. (2016). Fragranced consumer products: Exposures and effects from emissions. *Air Quality, Atmosphere & Health,* 9, 861–866.

Sunderland, E. M., et al. (2019). A review of the pathways of human exposure to poly- and perfluoroalkyl substances (PFASs). *Environmental Science & Technology,* 53(16), 9167–9185.

World Health Organization. (2013). *State of the Science of Endocrine Disrupting Chemicals.* WHO Press.

www.ingramcontent.com/pod-product-compliance
Lightning Source LLC
LaVergne TN
LVHW100522110826
845146LV00002B/746

9798218921200